A healthy hedonist's guide to...

LONDON

HIITB

WORKING OUT
IS THE NEW
GOING OUT...

A HEALTHY HEDONIST'S GUIDE TO LONDON

The ultimate guide for pleasure seekers in search of balance.

Do you want to know where to find the best workouts in London but also where to reward your efforts afterwards? Find your balance in this healthy hedonist's guide.

Focusing on six happening neighbourhoods, this guide is for pleasure seekers who are looking for ways to stay fit and healthy without missing out on London's vibrant scene.

DOSE is an online magazine for healthy hedonists. Sign up to receive the weekly newsletters

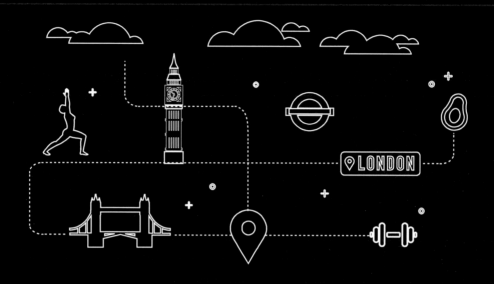

Sign up to receive the newsletters at
whateveryourdose.com

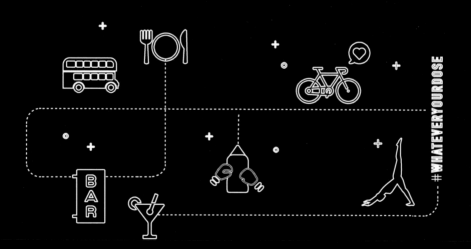

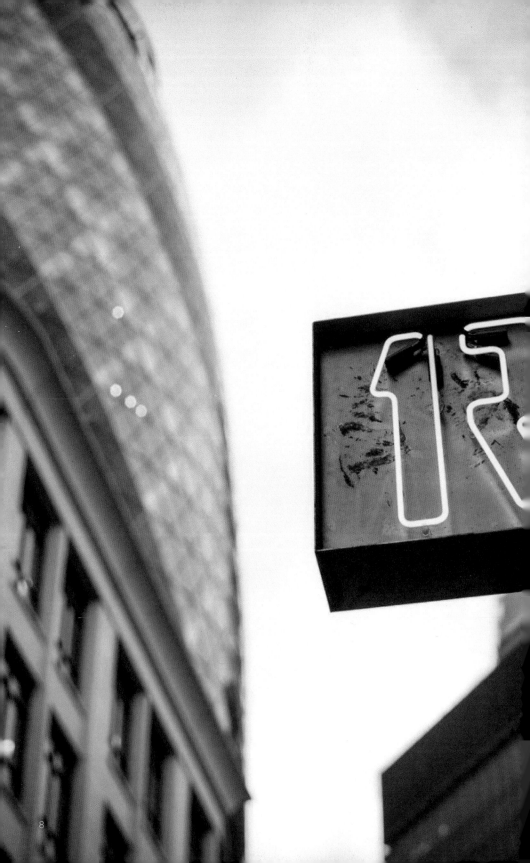

CITY & EAST

You might find yourself sipping a rainbow latte after working up a sweat in Hackney... walking from your class through the graffiti-filled streets of Shoreditch to a Bombay-style café... or squeezing in a fast and furious lunchtime workout in the heart of the City.

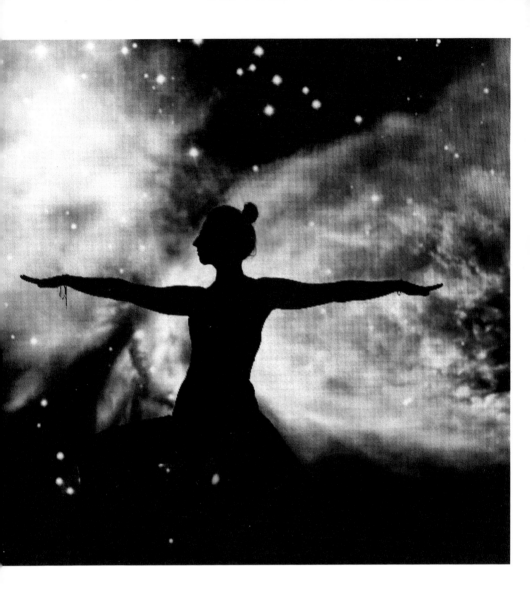

FLY LDN

YOGA | BARRE | TRX

If you like multi-sensory fitness experiences set to spine tingling playlists, you're going to love FLY LDN. Tap into unlimited zen at this studio in the heart of the City with beautifully crafted flows set to cinematic visuals (think, breathtaking Himalayan mountain ranges one minute and crashing ocean swells the next). Classes range from slow flows to more dynamic sequences designed to make you sweat, breathe deeper and focus your mind away from the city hustle. There's also a barre class built around music that draws on Pilates, yoga and dance to build core strength and improve balance, posture and flexibility. They use bodyweight, light weights, balls and resistance bands for intensity, variety and progression. Also on offer is an intense, low-impact class combining TRX-assisted stretching and Yoga to help you build strength and mobility. Leave your workout fully blissed out and reward efforts with healthy grub at POD and Tossed - both are within a 5 minute walk. For something more indulgent, head to Breakfast and Burgers or Swingers for a round of crazy golf, pizza and cocktails. Because it's about balance, right?

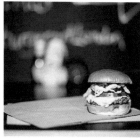 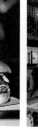 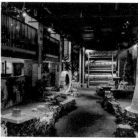 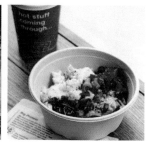

@BfastAndBurgers

@swingersldn

@tosseduk

📍 24 Creechurch Lane. London. EC3A 5EH

🚇 Tube: Aldgate (Circle, Hammersmith & City, Metropolitan)

Notes

....

....

....

....

....

....

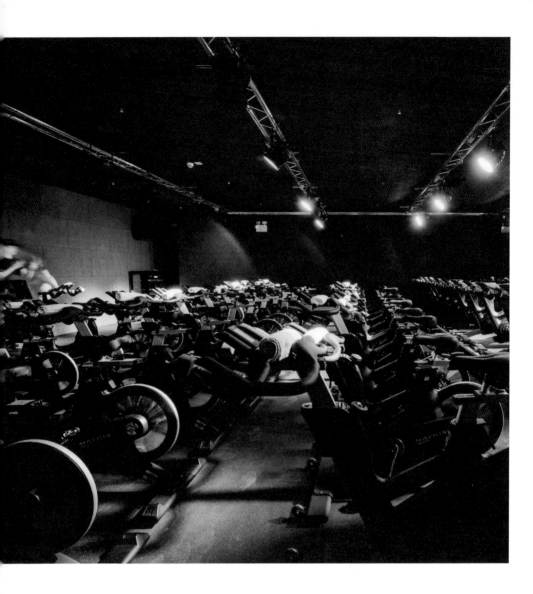

1REBEL

HIIT | INDOOR CYCLING | BOXING

1Rebel disrupted London's fitness club scene with its strobe-lit studios, thumping sound systems and euphoric playlists. It introduced us to a new form of going out, where we'd be hurtling through high-intensity training one minute, riding hard at 150mph the next. Sessions at the studio include Reshape - a half treadmill, half floor, 45-minute blast of physical and mental intensity. Whether you're looking to reshape the upper, lower or full body – there are classes for all. Mix it up with a 'Double Shot' – 30 minutes Reshape, 30 minutes Ride. Or why not choose a signature live session, featuring London's top DJs, Garage MCs and musicians from saxophonists to bongo drummers. If you prefer boxing to a beat, try 'Rounds' at their moody, underground lair beneath Broadgate Circle - less than a five minute walk away. Make use of the chilled scented towels and top of the range grooming amenities. Finish your session with an appointment with their in-house Barber + Blow dry bar or even raise a glass at the renowned 1R Prosecco Fridays. Grab a healthy bite to eat from Farmer J, The Good Yard or Tossed.

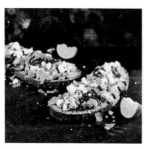
@farmerjfood

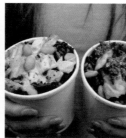
@tosseduk

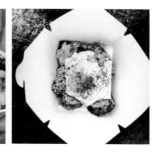
@goodyardldn

📍 **Address:** *(St Mary Axe) 63 St Mary Axe, London, EC3A 8LE (Broadgate) Broadgate Circle, London, EC2M 2QS*

🚇 **Tube:** *Liverpool Street (Central, Circle, Hammersmith & City & Metropolitan)*

Notes

....

....

....

....

....

....

🍴

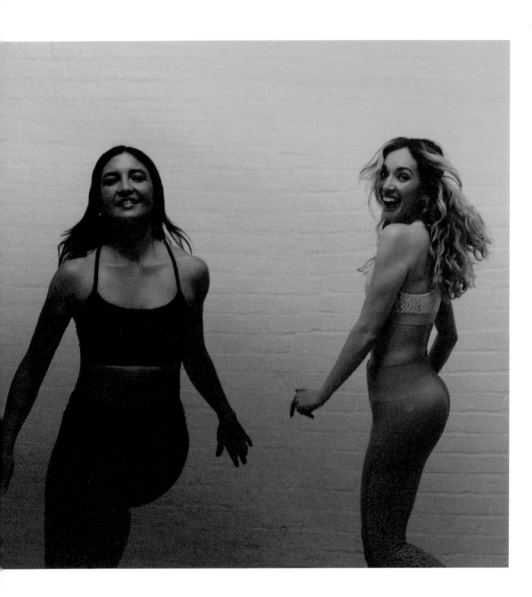

POP FIT

DANCE

Want to experience a workout from a dancer's perspective? Founded by former Royal Ballet School student Stephanie Burrows, Pop Fit offers three types of dance workouts: Signature – a full body conditioning class that borrows techniques from Pilates, yoga, plyometrics and dance, set to loud, fast, upbeat pop music. PlyoJam – that uses principles of plyometrics blended with dance moves and HIIT exercises, and Core – a low-impact workout choreographed to music and designed to work your core muscles. The beautifully designed sprawling facility features two studios, a breakout soft cushioned seating area, changing rooms with REN products and a retail capsule by Fabletics with a curated collection of ready-to-buy outfits and leggings. If it's a class and brunch affair, head to nearby Wringer & Mangle for poached eggs and a 'Green is God' smoothie. For evening sophistication, you're a ten minute walk from modern British restaurant Pidgin. If only wood oven pizza will do, visit Martello Hall for a slice of the Vegan Viking washed down with a bloody hot bloody Mary.

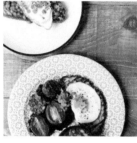
@wringerandmangle

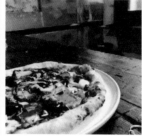
@martellohall

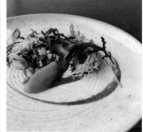
@pidginlondon

📍 *Address: 19 Sidworth Street, London Fields, London, E8 3SD*

🚇 *Tube: London Fields (Overground), Bethnal Green (Central)*

Notes

....

....

....

....

....

....

....

....

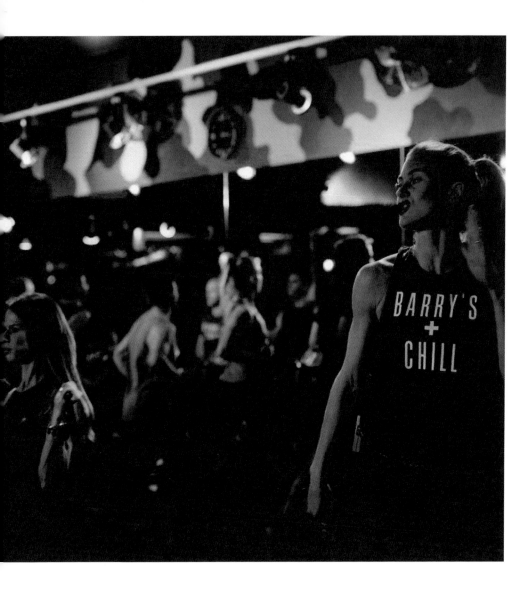

BARRY'S EAST

HIIT | STRENGTH & CONDITIONING

The boutique fitness market shows no sign of slowing down thanks to our penchant for cardio parties to bass-heavy pop music and a certain loud army-style bootcamp. The cult workout that fuses interval cardiovascular treadmill routines with strength training on the floor has grown into a veritable empire since its debut in 1998. This go-to workout for burning off steam (and shaving waistlines in the process) is still one of London's best-loved sweat fests with sell-out classes and memorable instructors. Whether you want to focus on Arms & Abs, Butt & Legs, Chest, Back & Abs, Core & Abs or the Full Body, there's a 60-minute class with your name on it. Prepare to work your socks off and be rewarded with a mighty endorphin rush. They don't call it the 'best workout in the world' for nothing. Shower off with Malin & Goetz products and swing by the on-site Fuel Bar for a grab and go protein smoothie. For dine in options, slip away to The Modern Pantry or Bad Egg for a breakfast of champions. For a rooftop meal with breathtaking views, head to The Aviary in Finsbury Square.

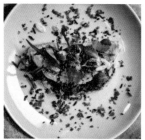 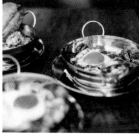 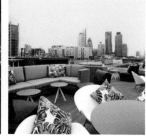

@themodernpantry   @the_baddest_egg   @aviaryldn

📍 **Address:** *2 Worship St, London, EC2A 2BH*

🚇 **Tube:** *Liverpool Street (Central, Circle, Hammersmith & City and Metropolitan lines)*

Notes

....

....

....

....

....

....

....

....

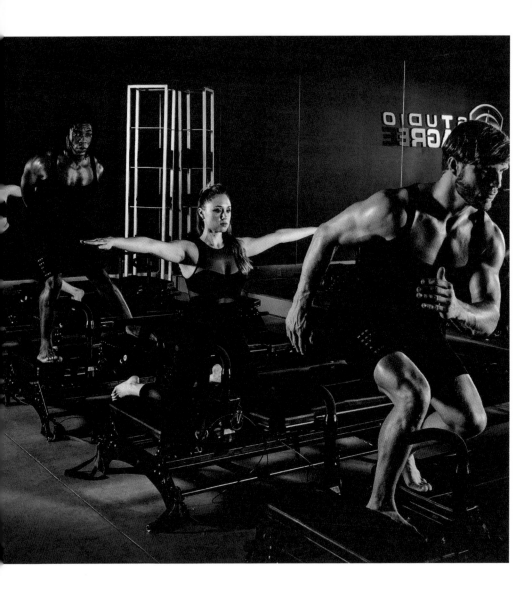

STUDIO LAGREE

PILATES

You pulse at the barre, stretch on the mat, sculpt on a reformer, and smash out some cardio in-between. But what if you could combine ALL of these moves in one workout? Enter Studio Lagree. The hottest workout from Hollywood, with studios in Toronto, Chicago, Munich and London, that tests your core, endurance, cardio, balance, strength and flexibility in every move. The signature M3 class will have you contorting your body on a sliding carriage similar to a reformer – except it's not a reformer at all, but a Megaformer. A highly evolved piece of kit with cut-outs and handles that allow you to make fast adjustments as you race through sets. Enter a heated, dimly-lit studio with a throbbing sound system and contort your body into the sort of positions that will work your muscles in ways you never thought possible. You'll be pouring with sweat in the first ten minutes with rounds of v-sits, lunges, squats and oh-so-many planks, to carve a killer core. Shower off and reward efforts at nearby Protein Haus, Beany Green, Benugo or POD.

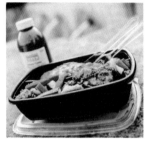 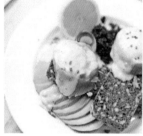 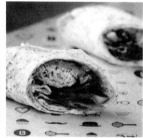

@proteinhaus

@beanygreen

@benugouk

 Address: *Studio Lagree, 35 Chiswell Street, London, EC1Y4SE*

Tube: *Moorgate (Hammersmith, Circle, Metropolitan, Northern), Old Street (Northern). Barbican (Hammersmith, Circle and Metropolitan)*

Notes

....

....

....

....

....

....

....

....

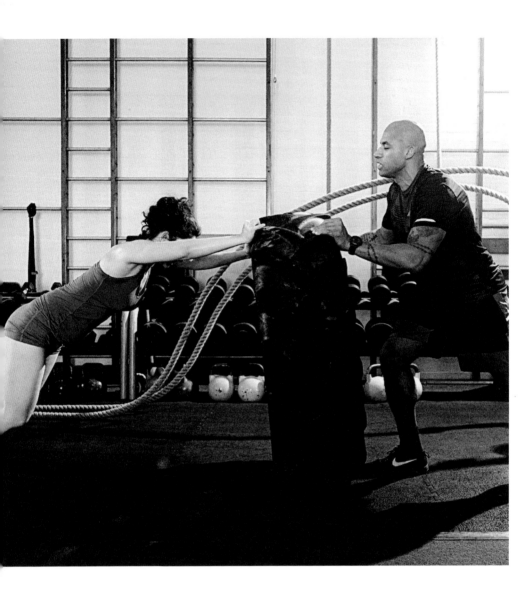

THE FOUNDRY

STRENGTH & CONDITIONING

Just a five minute walk from Old Street station, discover a results-driven gym where only the strong belong. If you're serious about pushing your fitness to the next level, it's time to build some proper foundations. This is where London's top instructors go to train. Discover cult classes such as City Strongman – known as one of the toughest workouts in the City. Find the same toys you'd expect to see in the World's Strongest Man circuit.

Only instead of record-breaking feats of strength, they use lighter loads for an effective fat-burning workout. Think: log lifting, sled dragging, prowler pushing and atlas stone carrying. If you fancy some HIIT, try SWEAT. A 45-minute class packed with challenging calisthenic movements, fusing circuits of strongman toys with Versa Climbers and Concept 2 rowers. Or if you're working towards a goal and classes aren't doing it for you, try a semi-private session instead. With a maximum 4 people, this is a great option for those who can't afford a PT but are looking for the same quality coaching and attention. As for post-workout plans, try some ceviche at a nearby Peruvian kitchen, grab something easy from Naughty Avocado or walk 10 minutes to Lantana Cafe for Buddha bowls and seriously punchy coffee.

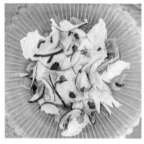
@cevicheuk

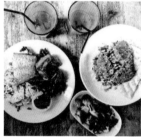
@lantanacafe

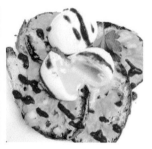
@naughtyavocado

Address: 227 City Rd, London, EC1V 1JT

Tube: Old Street (Northern)

Notes

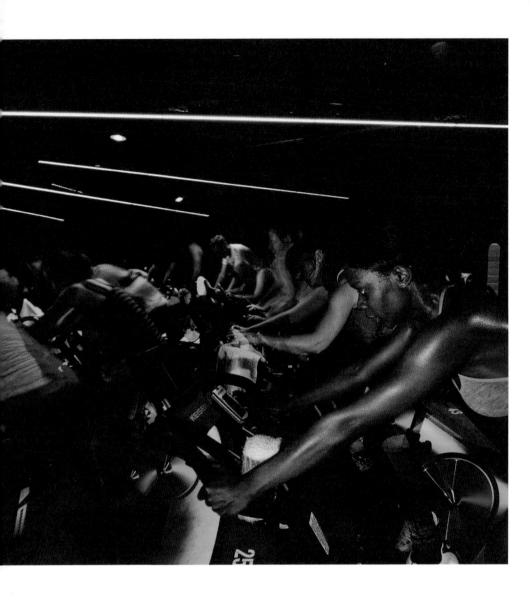

DIGME FITNESS

INDOOR CYCLING | HIIT

If you're a fan of competitive sports and video games, you'll fit in just fine at Digme, an immersive indoor cycling experience in Moorgate. Discover a dramatic, nightclub-style studio with theatre seating and colourful strobe lights. Climb aboard your Keiser M3i bike that tracks and measures data and clip in your cleats (complimentary shoes are provided). The instructor faces towards you on a stage and there's a large screen behind displaying a virtual road with a team of avatars cycling along a scenic route. We say team... but view each one as the enemy - this is a competition after all. Whilst they all look the same, the giveaway is your bike number that corresponds to an avatar on the screen. And a dreaded leaderboard that intermittently pops up during the class, displaying your efforts for all to see. A little healthy competition definitely helped us to work that

bit harder. But don't expend all your energy at once. This is all about stamina and endurance. Post class, you'll receive an email with a summary of your ride with information on mileage, calories, watts, cadence and RPM. Shower off with Cowshed products, and swing by the on-site cafe for a protein shake. Walk ten minutes to Simple Health Kitchen or treat yourself to a unique blend of Japanese, Brazilian, and Peruvian cuisine at SUSHISAMBA.

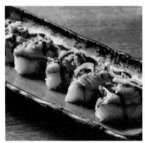 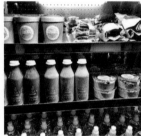 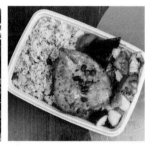

@sushisamba   @digmefitness   @simplehealthkitchen

📍 **Address:** *Moor Place (via Moor Lane), 1 Fore Street, London, EC2Y 5EJ (Other locations in Richmond, Blackfriars (HIIT classes available here) and Oxford Street)*

🚇 **Tube:** *Moorgate (Northern)*

Notes

....

....

....

....

....

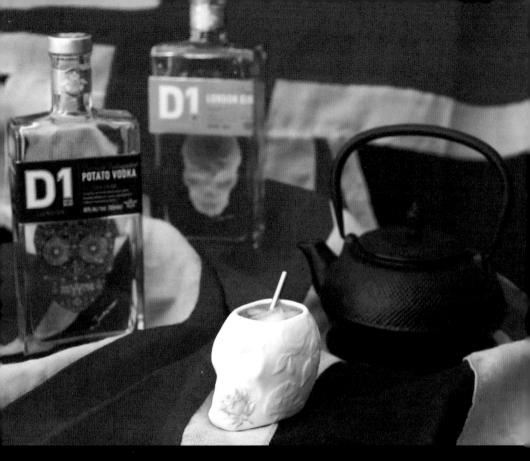

DI SPIRITS

D1 London Gin is a multi-award winning smooth and versatile gin which includes a daring kick of nettles that balances fruit flavours and aromas. The reversible bottle provides a clear canvas for the iconic 'Floral Skull', from the series of artworks by international artist Jacky Tsai, originally made famous by Alexander McQueen. D1 Potato Vodka is a spirit of outstanding character that combines delicious creamy smoothness with the diverse cultural references of Jacky Tsai's Stained Glass Skull.

D1 cocktail

30ml D1 London Dry Gin
15ml D1 Potato Vodka
30ml Green Tea
10ml Homemade Ginger Syrup
2 Dashes Bittermens Hopped
Grapefruit Bitters

Shake and fine strain into
Royal Crown Derby Skull
vessel over crushed ice.

NOBU SHOREDITCH

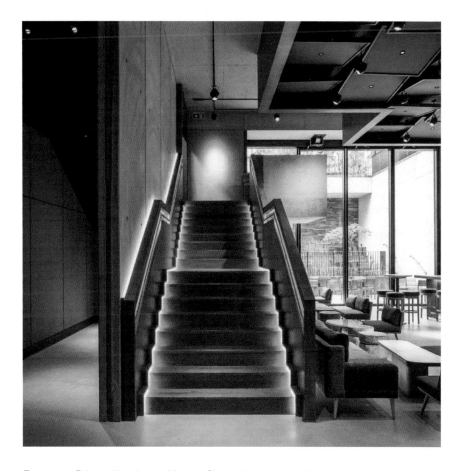

Enjoy a D1 cocktail at Nobu Shoreditch and dine on Yellowtail with Jalapeño and Wood Oven Roasted Lobster with Hakaido Scallops, Cilantro Aioli and Ikura. The stunning bar offers guests a sumptuous place to relax with friends and enjoy exquisite cocktails. In warmer months, escape to a garden oasis adjacent to the bar for a more intimate setting.

Address: 10-50 Willow Street, London, EC2A 4BH

Tube: Liverpool Street (Central)

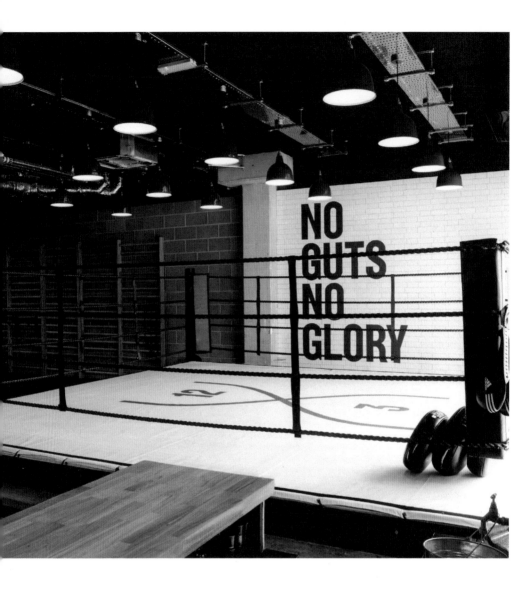

12 X 3 GYM

BOXING

Like Mickey Goldmill to Rocky Balboa, behind every fighter is a great coach. Whether you're new to boxing or competing for a title, you won't reach your potential without one. Find yours at 12 x 3 Gym in Aldgate. A boxing experience founded by Darren Barker and Ryan Pickard - sparring partners who met at Repton Boxing Club and went on to fight for club and country. Both were trained up by the legendary Tony Burns MBE so they understand the importance of a great coach and the special relationship you can build with them. Based on the signature workout of 12 x 3 minute rounds, the focus is on six key areas of training that are equally important to becoming a complete boxer: speed, stamina, strength, footwork, timing and mindset. With no big classes, you can choose from 1-to-1 training or a group session with a maximum class size of 4. The traditional boxing gym is home to old school techniques without complicated machinery or flashing lights. Anyone is welcome, so long as they have respect for the ring and a genuine desire to box. Post workout, head to Flavour Garden or Exmouth Coffee Company for a vegan apricot croissant.

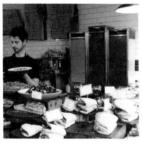 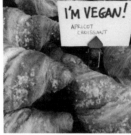 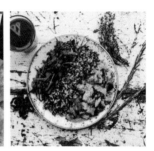

@exmouthcoffeecompany   @coppaclub   @flavour_garden

Address: 76 Alie Street, Aldgate, London, E1 8PZ (12 X 3 have another studio in Paddington)

Tube: Aldgate East (District, Hammersmith & City), Aldgate (Circle, Metropolitan)

Notes

....

....

....

....

....

....

....

....

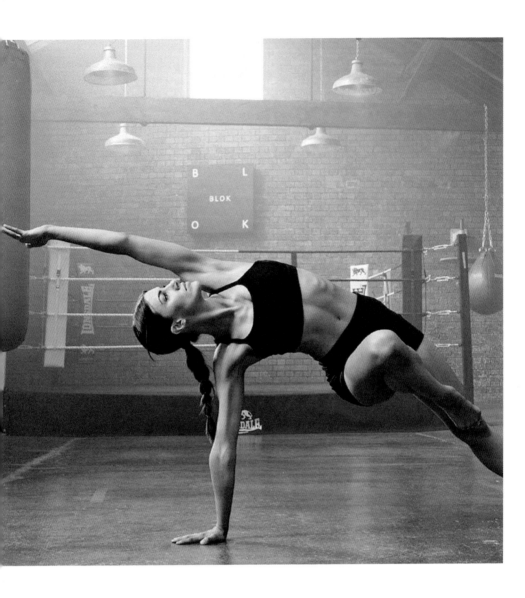

BLOK

BARRE | YOGA | HIIT

An industrial-style East London hangout with bare brick walls, vaulted concrete ceilings and cast iron pillars. Whether you're looking for dynamic or restorative, power yoga or yoga for beginners, Ashtanga or Yin, there are classes to suit a range of abilities. We're a fan of Blok Flow, a music-led sequence that bridges the gap between hardcore fitness and traditional yoga, created by renowned yogi and dance choreographer Ida May. Mix it up with strength and conditioning classes like Blok Fit, Functional Fitness, HIIT and Methodology X. There's also primal movement classes that incorporate crawls, hops, jumps, boxing, Pilates and barre. If you fancy something more playful for the weekend, rave your way to fitness with the aptly named 'Blok Party'. For post-workout grab and go refreshment, the in-house café offers a menu of sustainably sourced seasonal food to boost energy and fuel your workout. Peruse a selection of healthy, natural breakfast pots, protein pots and pre-prepared meals available to eat in or take away. The café also boasts the UK's first bone broth bar in a gym. If you're planning on heading out afterwards, make use of the showers and hairdryers. We recommend a post-workout brunch at Palm Vaults, one of London's most Instagrammable coffee haunts. Also try Lyle's and My Neighbour's the Dumplings.

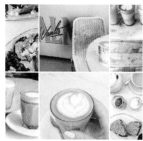 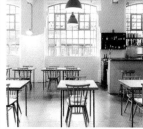 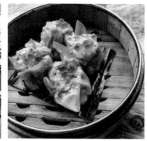

@palmvaults   @lyleslondon   @myneighboursthedumplings

Address: *Clapton Tram Depot, 38-40 Upper Clapton Road, E5 8BQ (BLOK has another studio in Shoreditch)*

Tube: *Clapton (Overground), Rectory Road (Overground)*

Notes

....

....

....

....

....

....

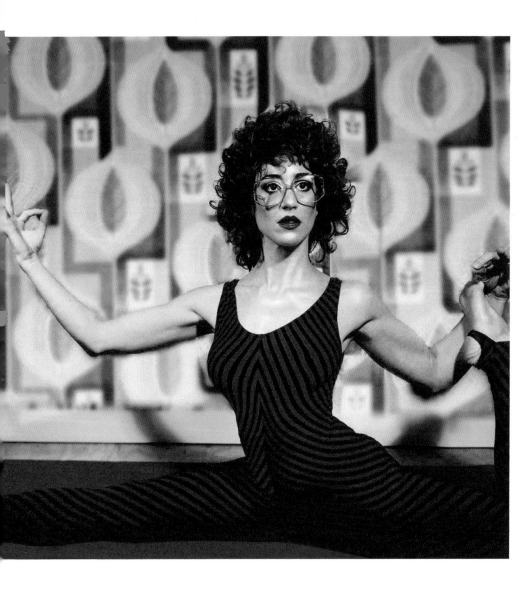

THE REFINERY

BARRE | YOGA | PILATES | DANCE

The art of refining, where unwanted substances are removed... be it weekend toxins or stale stagnant energy, switch it up for a dose of happiness at this fitness playground. Located in a sleekly designed underground bunker with tunnels, low ceilings and exposed concrete, classes range from mindfulness mediation and Yoga Fit Flow to R*U*S*H HIIT - a mash up of kettlebells, medicine balls, weight training and callisthenics to get you fitter and faster.

Other cult classes include 'Disco Barre' with Sophie Ritchie – a barre-based workout set to underground disco and house favourites, Derrier @ Haus of Barre9 – an intense barre-based conditioning workout, focusing on lifting the (you guessed it) and the aptly named Happy Hour @ The Barre where you can say 'cheers' to your body and make new friends sans hangover!

For some post-workout fuel, shower off and head to The Well Kitchen, a snug, independent cafe over the road serving great coffees and breakfasts (smashed avocado, baked eggs and beans, that sort of thing). Other great foodie spots in this area include The Grand Howl, Cafe Miami and Legs. For Michelin-starred dining, head to Pidgin.

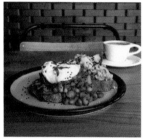
@the_grandhowl

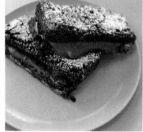
@_cafemiami

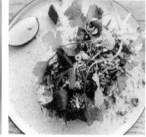
@legsrestaurant

Address: *14 Collent St, Hackney, London, E9 6SG*

Tube: *Hackney Central (Overground)*

Notes

....

....

....

....

....

....

....

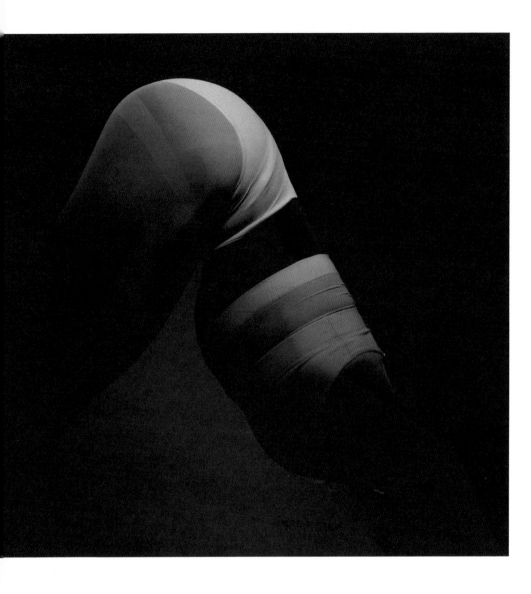

CHROMAYOGA

YOGA

An immersive yoga experience that combines light therapy, soundscapes and bespoke natural scents. The classes are simply titled: Red, Orange, Pink, Blue and Yellow, each promising a full spectrum of benefits, designed around mood. Red for energy. Blue to reset the natural circadian rhythms and aid sleep disorders such as winter depression (S.A.D) and Yellow to aid digestion and mood swings. We don't know about you but we think we could benefit from the full spectrum. In each class, the teacher guides you through a set of sequences that correspond to the healing properties of that colour, set to a specially composed soundtrack that emulates the frequencies our brains emit in different states of consciousness. Essential oils have also been developed to correspond with each class colour. These scents are used in harmony with yoga poses to drive energy, aid breath work, release muscle tension and encourage relaxation. As well as providing an immersive yoga experience, their approach to wellbeing uses many techniques off the mat. A team of in-house practitioners offer advice on how to balance your body on the inside and provide a range of treatments from acupuncture to herbal tonics which can aid many common physical and emotional issues. Grab a bite to eat afterwards at Hoxton Grill, The Breakfast Club, Lantana Cafe, or Ozone.

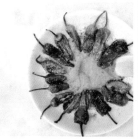 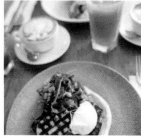 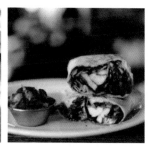

@hoxtongrill　　　　*@lantanacafe*　　　　*@thebrekkyclub*

 Address: *45 Charlotte Rd, London, EC2A 3DP*

Tube: *Old Street (Northern), Liverpool Street (Central, Circle, Hammersmith & City, Metropolitan)*

Notes

....

....

....

....

....

....

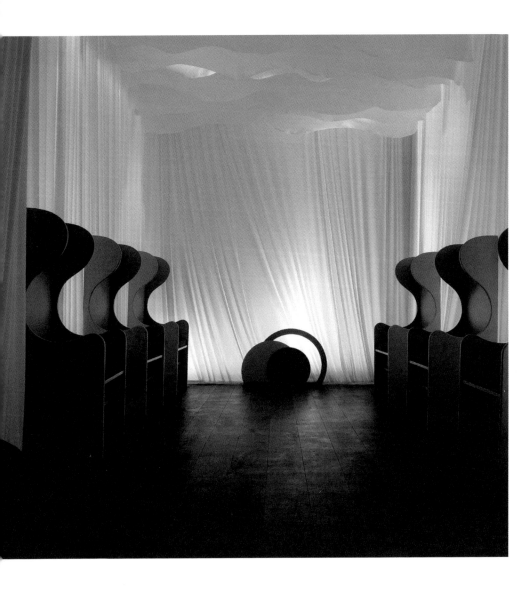

INHERE STUDIO

MEDITATION

We don't think twice about booking classes that rev us up, but what about ones that wind us down? Try switching off occassionally, it will do wonders for your productivity and this one you can even do in a suit. Inhere is a drop-in meditation studio in the heart of the City. Choose between 20, 30 and 40-minute sessions that fit with the flow of your day. Whether you're looking for a centred start, a reset at lunch or a gentle unwind after work... sit down in one of nine meditation spaces – six chairs or three floor seats, and be lulled into a calm, meditative state by soothing soundscapes. You'll be guided through breathing and mindfulness techniques, before being brought back to the real world with sound and lighting. Book a seat via their app, or drop in. Once the session starts, you can't disturb others by allowing late entry, so arrive at least five minutes early to get settled. If you think the whole office could benefit from some time out, book a corporate wellbeing package. The centre also has a Crussh café if you'd like to pick up breakfast or lunch when you visit, or try Hummus Bros or Protein Haus.

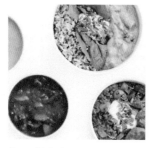 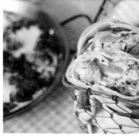 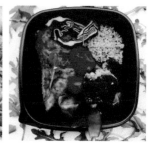

@crusshjuicebars   @hummus_bros   @proteinhausuk

📍 **Address:** *Light Centre in Monument, 36 St Mary at Hill, London EC3R 8DU*

🚇 **Tube:** *Monument (Circle & District)*

Notes

....

....

....

....

....

....

....

....

....

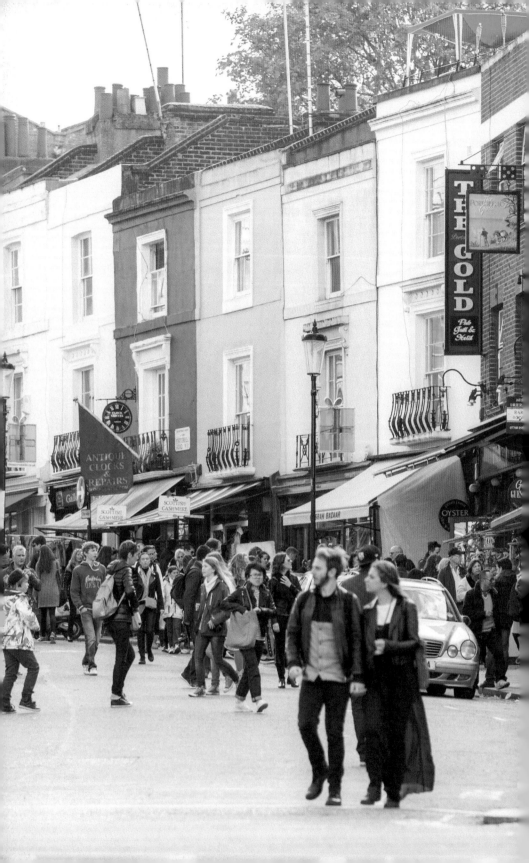

WEST

Find HIIT workouts disguised as games in Hyde Park, brunch spots aplenty in Westbourne Grove, bustling markets in Portobello and a gritty, raw and very real boxing gym in Ladbroke Grove (David Beckham is a fan!)

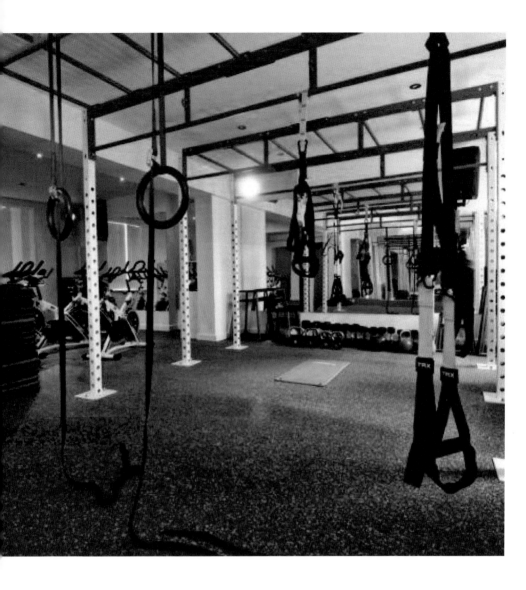

GYM CLASS

HIIT | STRENGTH

If you're lucky enough to live in Holland Park, or even on its outskirts (otherwise known as Shepherd's Bush), the chances are you're less bothered about its rich horticulturalist past and more concerned with where to be seen in your activewear. Head to Gym Class for a super-charged workout fusing cardio and resistance training where you can work hard through sequences of burpees, lunges, squats, tyre flipping and battle ropes. Try GUNS N' GLUTES

- a hardcore workout designed to get the week off to a roaring start, combining full body HIIT and strength moves. Pick up a protein shake, fresh juice or snack from reception. There's limited changing facilities here, so you might want to think about going home first before heading somewhere fancy like Casa Cruz just a few doors down. You're also within a 10 minute walk of Westfield Shopping Centre with fast food favourites like Itsu, LEON and Tossed. Or why not make a day of it and head to Cowshed Clarendon Cross for post-workout Bellinis and Avocado & Eggs before hitting the spa.

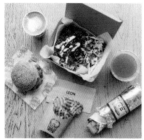
@leonrestaurants

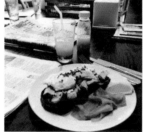
@cowshed

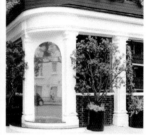
@casacruzlondon

📍 **Address:** Gym Class, 45 Phillimore Walk, Holland Park, W8 7RZ

🚇 **Tube:** Holland Park (Central)

Notes

....

....

....

....

....

....

....

....

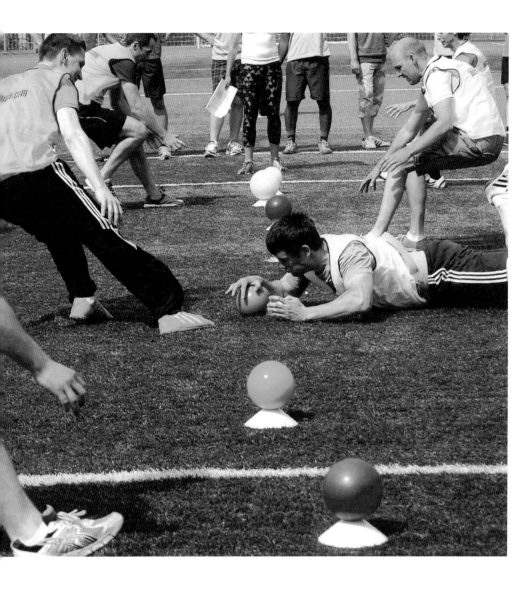

RABBLE

OUTDOOR FITNESS

The brainchild of former athlete Charlotte Roach, who after suffering a terrible injury got back on her bike and cycled from Beijing to London (as you do...) to raise money for the air ambulance that saved her life. She then went on to set up her own business, Rabble. High-intensity training disguised as games from British Bulldogs to Dodgeball, designed to make fitness fun, engaging, enjoyable, varied and social. You'll be so busy trying to work out the strategy that you'll forget you're actually undertaking fitness drills and because these games are team-based you will make some great friends along the way. Find Rabble games in various locations including Hyde Park. For post-workout refreshment head to the Serpentine Kitchen for brunch and if you're feeling brave, a refreshing dip in The Lido. Or if only a pub will do... pay a visit to The Mall Tavern, The Champion or The Churchill and treat yourself to some well-earned grub and a frothing pint.

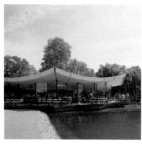 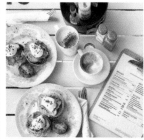 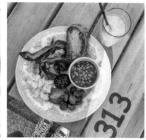

@serpentinekitchen *@serpentinekitchen* *@supamike08*

Address: *Rabble Games, 77-83 Park Ln, Mayfair, London, W1K 7HB*

Tube: *Queensway (Central), Hyde Park Corner (Piccadilly)*

Notes

....

....

....

....

....

....

....

....

....

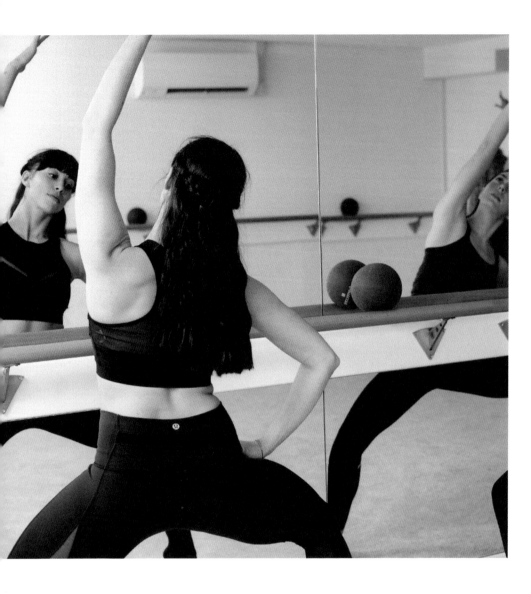

BARRECORE

BARRE

Recognised as London's original Barre studio with locations all across the City. Inspired by the moves of ballet, Pilates, yoga and functional training, Barrecore's signature squeezing, pulsing isometric stretches will leave you with a clear head and killer core. In the heart of bustling Kensington, find this studio just across the road from Sweaty Betty, opposite St. Mary Abbots Church. Ring the buzzer for entry. Classes include barrecoreMIXED, a low impact full body interval training program using isometric exercises alternated with stretching to create a long, lean physique. Prefer your workout to a beat? Try barrecoreASANA that incorporates the signature barre moves to uplifting music to get you mentally centered for the day ahead. Or if you want to crank it up some more, try barreSCULPT with resistance bands for added intensity! After all that sculpting, shower and head to the cosy, ecclectic Maggie Jones (they love dogs here) or Crussh for some grab and go fitness food. You're also within walking distance of London's flagship Whole Foods, that boasts three floors overflowing with all the flavours you could wish for in one place — including an entire floor dedicated to eat-in options.

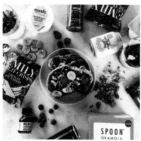
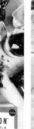
@wholefoodsuk

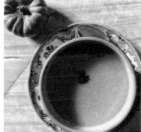
@maggiejonesrestaurant

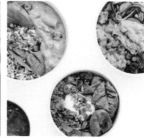
@crusshjuicebars

Address: *18 Kensington Church Street, London, W8 4EP*

Tube: *High Street Kensington (Circle & District)*

Notes

....

....

....

....

....

....

....

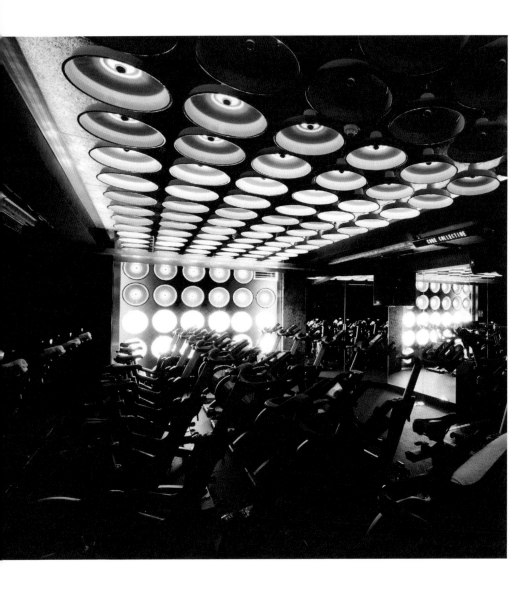

CORE COLLECTIVE

HIIT | YOGA | STRENGTH | PILATES | INDOOR CYCLING

If you like to mix it up, look no further than Core Collective in High Street Kensington that serves up a mighty blend of high Intensity interval training, power yoga, TRX, rowing, mat Pilates, indoor cycling and classes for active recovery. This stylish, contemporary space that's part health food cafe, part fitness lair is a true playground for fitness junkies. The industrial luxe aesthetic will also look fabulous on your Instagram feed. Try 'Cycle' - 45 minutes of endurance cycling in a basement nightclub with a throbbing sound system and Tron-style lighting. Lose yourself as you push through the climb, saddle up in the sprint and move to the beat of expertly curated playlists. Post-workout, reward efforts at the CC kitchen serving up Aussie-style eggs, Ozone coffee and wholesome salad boxes. If you fancy a change of scene, try Café Phillies over the road or The Ivy Kensington Brasserie.

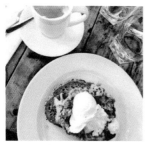
@cafephillies

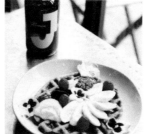
@corecollectivekitchen

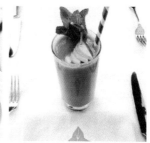
@theivykensington

📍 *Address: 45 Phillimore Walk, Holland Park W8 7RZ*

🚇 *Tube: High Street Kensington (Circle & District)*

Notes

....

....

....

....

....

....

....

....

....

....

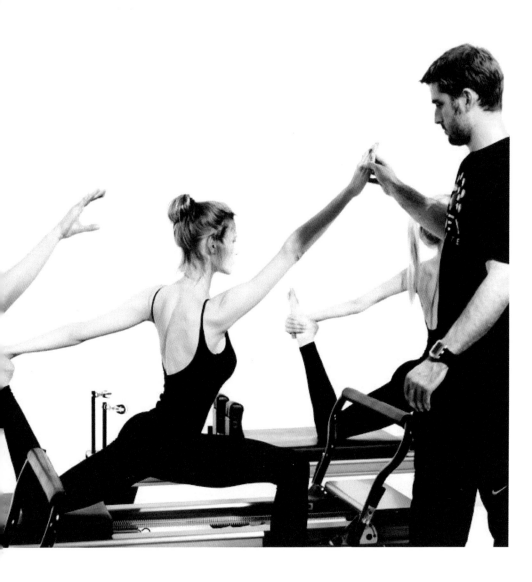

TEN HEALTH & FITNESS

PILATES | PHYSIO | BARRE | HIIT

A few minutes from Ladbroke Grove, this light, bright Notting Hill studio offers a full breadth of stretch and sculpting services. As Ten's HQ, it's also their biggest set-up, with three studios, three therapy rooms and a gym. Classes here include: Pilates for beginners, intermediate and advanced. Jumpboard, Prenatal and Cardiolates, HIIT, TenRX, Barre and Personal Training. If you're tired of smashing HIIT classes and pounding pavements, this studio that focusses on injury prevention, is for you. Book in for a full Body MOT service - great for anyone who has a recurring niggle, or is thinking of taking up a new sport. It's also a good way to check for any underlying issues or predisposition to injury, whether as part of your lifestyle, your work set-up, or from a postural imbalance. Try a session with Cheyne Voss, Ten's Head of Physiotherapy and the go-to physio of top athletes, actors and models. For post workout refreshment head to Snaps & Rye or Lowry & Baker, both are within a 10 minute walk.

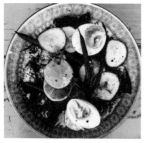 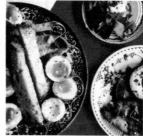 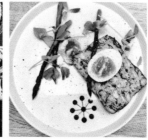

@lowryandbaker   *@lowryandbaker*   *@snapsandrye*

📍 **Address:** *Ten Health & Fitness, 2-4 Exmoor Street, London, W10 6BD*

🚇 **Tube:** *Ladbroke Grove (Circle, Hammersmith & City)*

Notes

....

....

....

....

....

....

....

....

....

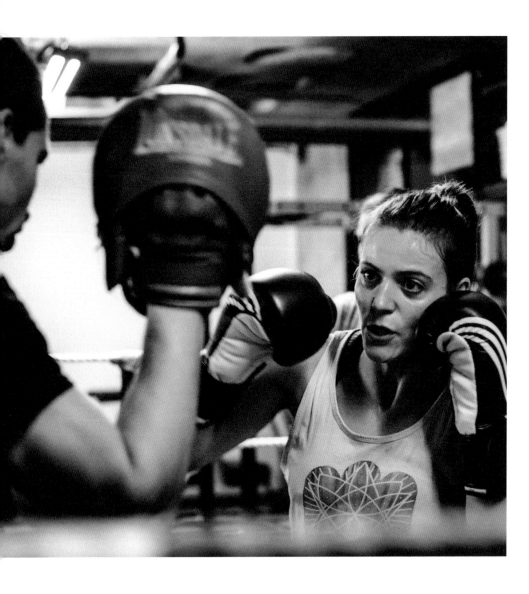

BOX CLEVER SPORTS

BOXING

The first rule of Fight Club is: you do not talk about Fight Club. The second rule of Fight Club is... you simply have to discover this hidden gem of a boxing gym. David Beckham is a fan. Set in a disused car park in Ladbroke Grove, find no shiny studio, optic lights and nightclub vibes but a gritty, raw and very real boxing gym, reminiscent of Tyler Durden's underground lair. Kick start your day with a 'Wake Up' session - a combination of boxing drills, cardio, bag work and an intense abs circuit, or finish the day with KO in one of their evening classes. If you want to improve boxing skills, try a non-contact 'Box Technical' session or to release that inner Rocky in you, go for 'Box Clever' with skipping, shadow boxing, bags, pad work and functional full body circuits. We love Pete Liggins' Saturday Morning Blitz – a tough, explosive, high energy class that'll make you earn a seriously good breakfast. Head to Bodyism's cafe for protein pancakes and a Body Brilliance shake. For lunch/dinner plans head to The Electric on Portobello Road or Peyotito for a serious Mexican feast. But be warned, there are no showers at Box Clever (it is located inside a car park - after all) so head home to shower before going out or prepare to sit sweaty in your kit.

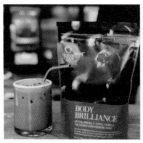
@bodyism

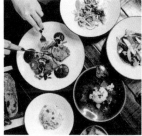
@peyotitolondon

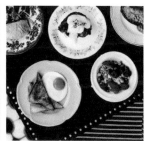
@electricdiner

📍 **Address:** *351 Westbourne Park Rd, Lowerwood Court Car Park, W11 1EU*

🚇 **Tube:** *Ladbroke Grove (Circle, Hammersmith & City)*

Notes

....
....
....
....
....
....
....

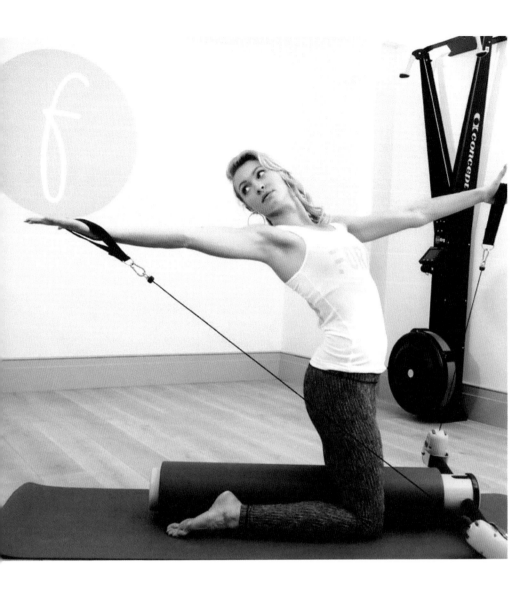

FORM STUDIOS

PILATES

Located on the corner of Portobello, this bijoux boutique became an instant hit with the West London crowd, and has garnered many a Tatler Gym Award in its time. The Pilates based, high-intensity class centres around the MOTR – half reformer, half foam roller that you can lie on, stand on and kneel on while using resistance bands in a range of movements.

The brainchild of celebrity trainer Elissa El Hadj, the workout blends the agility, lengthening and toning of Pilates with a surge of high-intensity called "the SPEED 8" – a circuit blast of SkiErg (a Nordic skiing simulator, a bit like rowing standing up), TRX and Kettlebells. Other classes include BOX-FIT, a full-on dynamic boxing class that mixes body weight exercises, shadow boxing and heavy bag work. FORM HIIT - a high-intensity interval training workout, with body weight movements, kettlebells, ski ergs, TRX and MOTR bars for fat-burning. Be warned, grippy or Pilates socks are essential. Complete your workout with a visit to Farmacy, Jusu Brothers, NAMA Foods or Bucket for seafood by the Bucketful - all within a 10 minute walk.

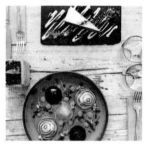
@namafoods

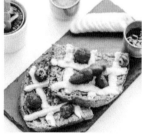
@jusubrothers

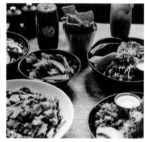
@farmacyuk

Address: 77 Lonsdale Rd, Notting Hill, London, W11 2DF

Tube: Bayswater (Circle & District) Notting Hill (Central, Circle & District)

Notes

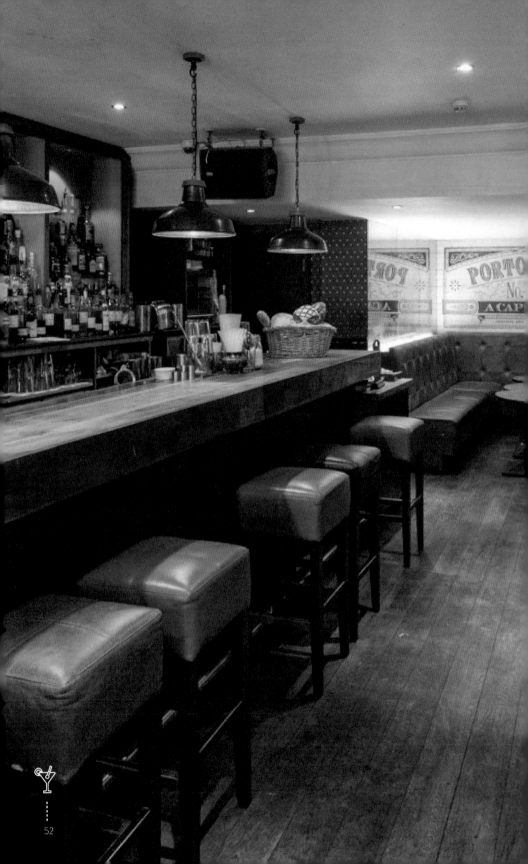

PORTOBELLO STAR

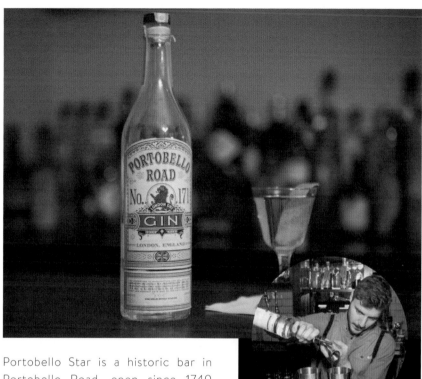

Portobello Star is a historic bar in Portobello Road, open since 1740 it has served drinks to the likes of royals, beggars, scarlet ladies, drunkards, intellectuals, popular musicians of the day, and now just the cool, fun crowd of Notting Hill. Immerse yourself in the stylish surroundings of Portobello's famous market while sipping on a gin cocktail.

Tip: Book a Ginstitute experience

Address: *171 Portobello Road, London, W11 2DY*

Tube: *Notting Hill Gate (Central, Circle & District)*

'The Queen Mother' Cocktail

25mls Portobello Road Gin
25mls Dubonnet
20mls Aperol
5mls Dark Jamaican Rum

Stir the ingredients with ice in a mixing glass or jug. Strain into a stemmed cocktail glass. Garnish with a twist of lemon and orange.

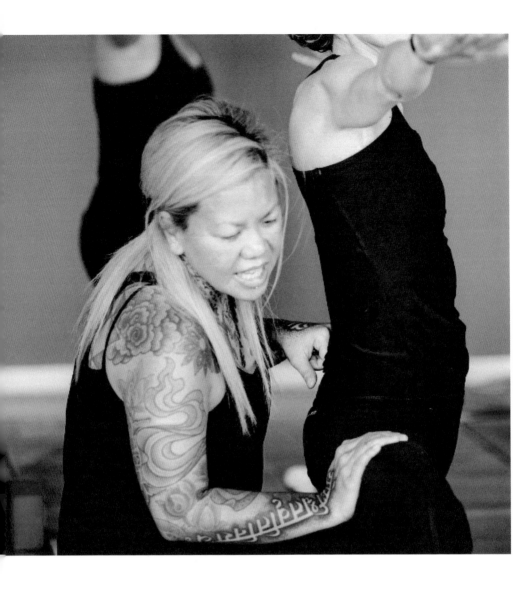

SANGYE YOGA

YOGA

From 'Sang' meaning 'awakening' from the sleep of ignorance and Gyé meaning 'opening' like a blossoming lotus flower to knowledge and wisdom - go on a journey of self-discovery at this Jivamukti studio in Kensal Rise. The yoga classes here are vigorously physical and you can expect some chanting, Yogic philosophical teachings and meditation woven in. Try a class with Melody Hekmat - a disciple of yoga gurus David Life and Sharon Gannon, who will entrance you with her heartfelt, nurturing classes and lashings of tiger balms. To keep the practice inspiring, asana sequences are ever-changing except for the signature Jivamukti class called Spiritual Warrior, which is a set sequence. The centre also hosts workshops, lectures and performances by internationally renowned teachers and artists. If you like mixing health with a little hedonism, head over to Paradise By Way of Kensal Rise. An award-winning restaurant and one of London's favourite nightclubs.

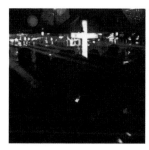
@paradisekensal

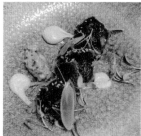
@paradisekensal

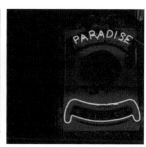
@paradisekensal

Address: *300 Kensal Rd, London, W10 5BE*

Tube: *Westbourne Park (Circle, Hammersmith & City)*

Notes

....

....

....

....

....

....

....

....

....

....

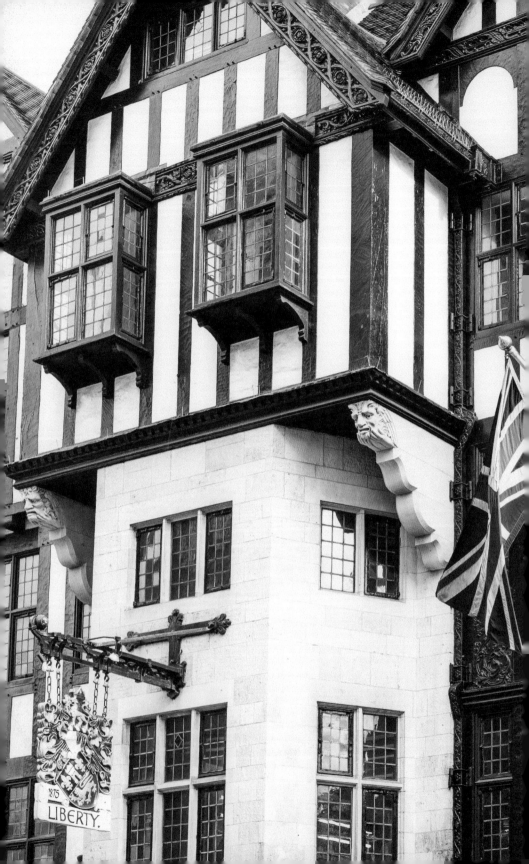

CENTRAL

Join a team of rockstar instructors for a party on a bike... find your zen at a yoga bar and bounce back with a vegan burger in Marylebone... or don your leg warmers and leotards in Victoria for dancing to 80's beats

SETTE VIE

The roots of Sette Vie Amaretto originate from a family of master distillers who have been perfecting their craft from the 1880's to today. This family, based in Abruzzo, Italy, began selling Amaretto under their own label in the late nineteenth century. As the recipe passed from father to son, the flavour profile has been refined while adhering to the family ethos of using only the best natural ingredients of the region. Sette Vie Amaretto is and always will be faithful to the rules set out by this family of Italian artisans.

Sette Vie cocktail

30ml Sette Vie Amaretto
15ml Sette Vie Melonchello
40ml Cloudy Apple Juice
15ml Lemon Juice

Shake and fine strain into an
Old Fashioned Rocks glass
over a large cube of ice.

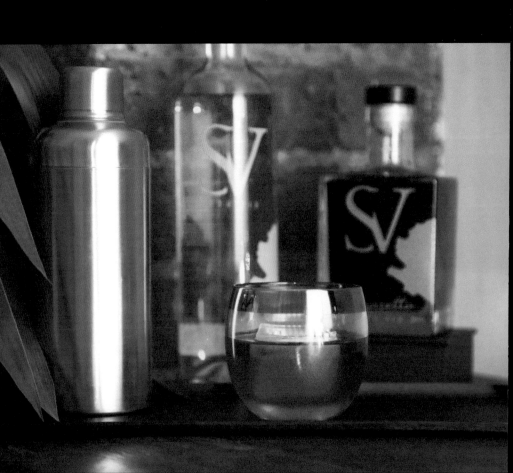

HOLBORN DINING ROOM

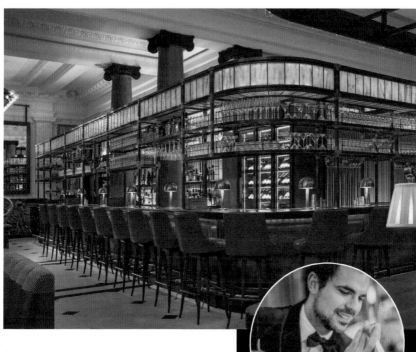

A vibrantly bustling salon that combines reclaimed oak with antique mirrors, red leather banquettes with tweed detailing. Home to 550 different gins and 27 tonics, it's a place for enjoying a convivial meal and a sophisticated tipple with friends.

Tip: Order 'La Folie Douce' at Holborn Dining Room's Gin Bar. Ask for Vitor Lourenço.

- -

📍 **Address:** *Holborn Dining Room, No. 252 High Holborn, London, WC1V 7EN*

🚇 **Tube:** *Holborn (Central)*

- -

La Folie Douce

G'Vine Florasion - 50ml
Vermouth Royal Rouge - 25ml
Red Currant Syrup - 20ml
Sette Vie Aperitivo - 10ml
Fresh lime juice - 10ml
Cherry bitters - 2 dashes

Shake all ingredients.
Double strain.

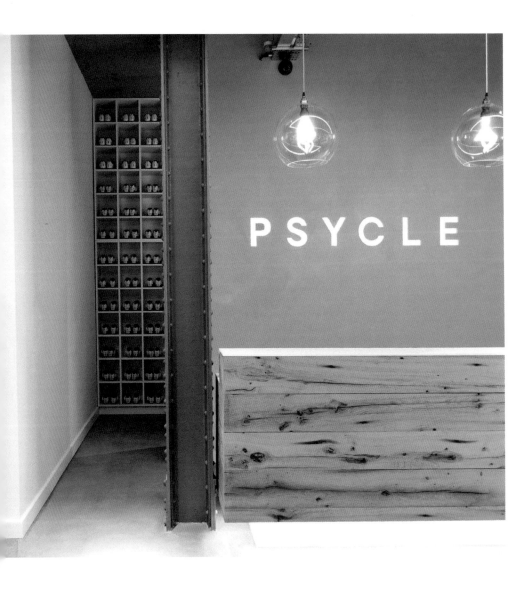

PSYCLE

INDOOR CYCLING

A full body physical and spiritual workout experience on a bike in a nightclub-style environment with neon strobes and booming beats. Expect to leave feeling uplifted and positively psyched for the day ahead. The high-energy classes run from early mornings right through to the evening, with 45, 60 & 90 minute classes designed to fit in with busy schedules suitable for any fitness level. We recommend a class with professional dancer, singer / songwriter and producer, A.D. His passion for music shines through in his goosebump-tingling playlists that will get you through those tough moments and get you feeling invigorated. Listen to his playlist before class to see if you feel his rhythm! Swing by the Energy Kitchen on exit for a nutritious juice or smoothie. For post-workout fuel, Fitzrovia is bursting with delights from Workshop Coffee next door, to Kaffeine, Maple & Fitz and Riding House Cafe.

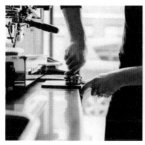
@workshopcoffee

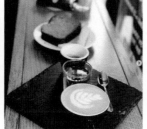
@kaffeinelondon

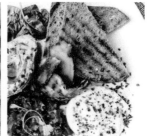
@mymapleandco

📍 **Address:** *76 Mortimer Street, London, W1W 7SA*

🚇 **Tube:** *Oxford Circus (Victoria, Central and Bakerloo)*

Notes

....

....

....

....

....

....

....

....

....

....

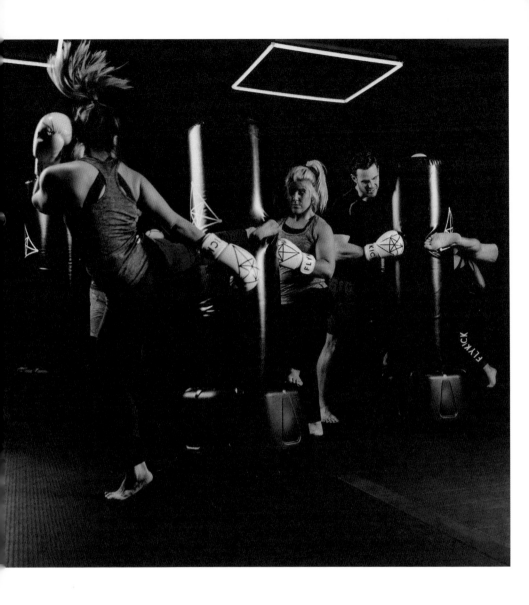

FLYKICK

KICKBOXING

You've tried boxing, in fact, you've perfected your one-twos and your footwork is a sight to behold. If you've become hooked on the benefits of boxing, from cardio fitness to confidence, stamina to strength, then you might want to check out Flykick, a boutique fitness studio that combines kickboxing-inspired training on a bag with a serious HIIT session and some stretching inbetween. The

5,000 square ft. studio boasts multiple instructors for each of its classes, ensuring everyone gets what they need out of the workout. Whether you've never thrown a punch before or your roundhouse kicks are enough to make Jean-Claude Van Damme green with envy, this studio is open for all. The workout – dubbed the 'Flykick Formula' – takes you through an all-encompassing, full-body HIIT circuit with all your favourite moves. Just when you think you can't sweat any more, you'll get a little active recovery while working on mobility before you glove up. Then, the fun really starts; on the bag you'll work through your jabs, crosses, hooks and uppercuts, as well as front and roundhouse kicks. Make use of the showers then reward efforts at Beany Green or Black Sheep Coffee in Regent's Place or try Mile 27 round the corner.

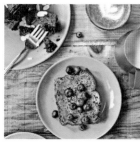
@beanygreen

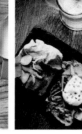
@black_sheep_coffee

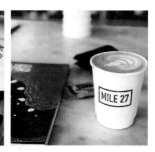
@miletwenty7

Address: *350 Euston Rd, London, NW1 3AX*

Tube: *Great Portland Street (Circle, Hammersmith & City)*

Notes

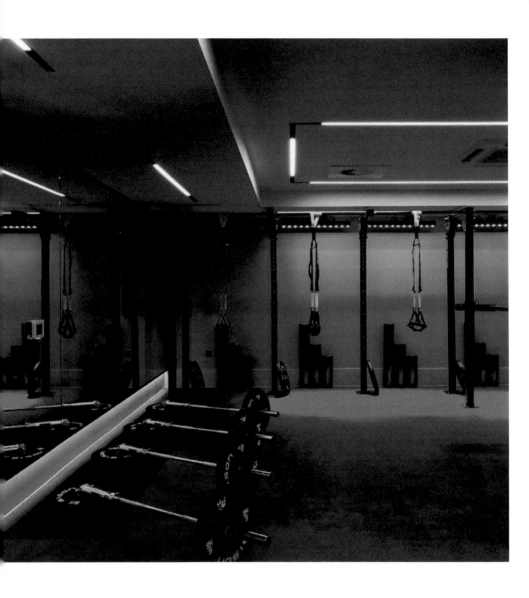

SWEAT BY BXR

BOXING | STRENGTH | CARDIO | YOGA

Whether you sweat for a beach snap or brunch, head over to this pay-to-train boutique round the corner from The Chiltern Firehouse to do it in style. With state-of-the-art lighting and a nightclub-grade sound system, an hour at this swanky facility is sure to get your heart racing and blood pumping. Try a blast of cardio on a Versa climber - a low-impact machine that feels a little like rowing standing up. A total body workout with a mixture of muscle isolations and intervals - some say it's the new spinning. Improve your boxing technique in the 'Skills' studio with a variety of drills from jabs, hooks and uppercuts to footwork. If you're looking to take your flexibility to the next level, whether it's progressive, ballistic or static, the 'Mobility' classes will develop the muscles to maximum effectiveness. Post class swing by Joe & The Juice, Natural Kitchen or Opso, or visit Yeotown Kitchen for a vegan burger, fries and a side of zen.

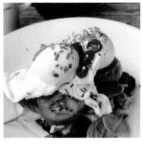 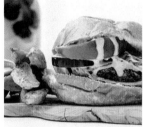 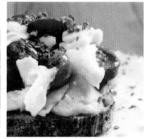

@naturalkitchen_london   @yeotownkitchen   @opso_london

📍 **Address:** *24 Paddington St, Marylebone, London, W1U 5QX*

🚇 **Tube:** *Baker Street (Bakerloo, Circle, Hammersmith & City, Jubilee, Metropolitan), Bond Street (Central, Jubilee), Marylebone (Bakerloo)*

Notes

....

....

....

....

....

....

....

....

....

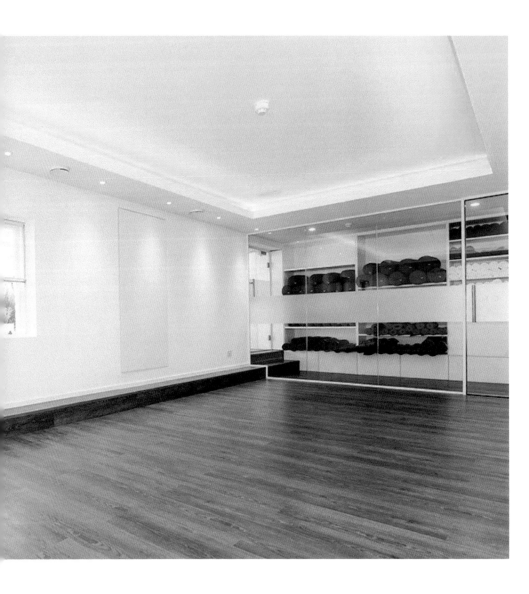

TOTAL CHI

YOGA | PILATES | MEDITATION

Just a three minute walk from Baker Street station and Regent's Park, find a serene garden studio decked with gongs, plants and Buddha statues, where you can unleash your inner zen. Listen to the tranquil sounds from a garden waterfall as you melt into a practice whether it's a dynamic Ashtanga, deep Iyengar, calming Hatha or flowing Vinyasa. Inside there are two studios that can be heated to 29 - 32 degrees C for warmer classes. Coloured LED's merge with natural daylight from the courtyard for a truly unique urban retreat. Melt into a slow, meditative Yin class or squeeze in a 45-minute Reformer Pilates class to get your lunchtime adrenaline fix. Cool off with a luxury rain shower using Malin & Goetz products and swing by the 'Yoga bar' for a healing juice, smoothie, birch water or turmeric mylk. Other foodie spots in this area include Saint Espresso and Fucina.

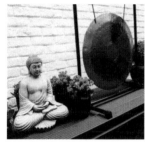
@totalchiyoga

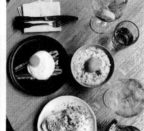
@fucinalondon

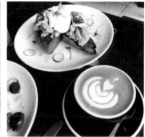
@saintespresso

Address: *243 Baker Street, Marylebone, London, NW1 6XE*

Tube: *Baker Street (Bakerloo, Jubilee)*

Notes

....

....

....

....

....

....

....

....

....

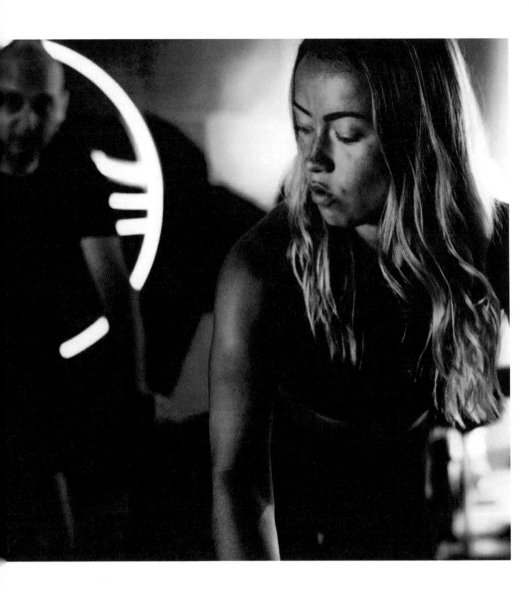

ONE 10

INDOOR CYCLING | HIIT

Baker Street may be synonymous with a certain pipe-smoking detective, but it's also home to hardcore, high-energy spinning. Motivational quotes are plastered along the stairwell to get you ready for the gruelling class ahead. The two studios are finished to a very high standard and are kitted out with smartbikes that keep track of your stats and class performance. There are two cycle classes to choose from: 'Nirvana' - a party-style ride with great music and choreography, and 'Paceline' for the more competitive types with endurance intervals designed to make you stronger for longer, hill climbs to improve your lactate threshold and power intervals that will push you to smash any sprint finishes! By the end you'll feel like you've finished a particularly hilly stage of the Tour de France. If want to take it up a notch try Threshold - a HIIT treadmill workout that tests speed, endurance and strength. Shower off with Cowshed products and head to Simple Health Kitchen next door, Vital Ingredient or Souli.

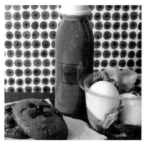
@simplehealthkitchen

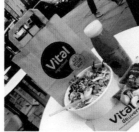
@vitalingredient

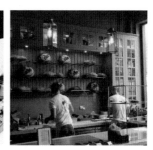
@soulifood

Address: 16 Baker Street, Marylebone, London, W1U 3HS

Tube: Baker Street (Bakerloo, Circle & District)

Notes

....

....

....

....

....

....

....

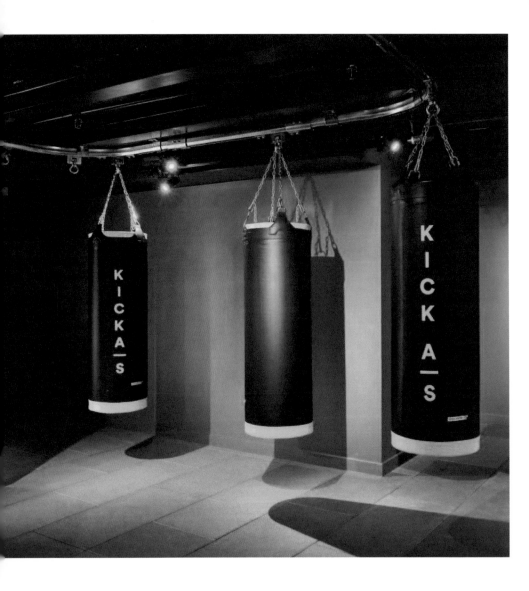

ANOTHER_SPACE

STRENGTH | HIIT | YOGA

Mix up your workouts at Another_Space – sister club to luxury members gym, Third Space. As London's nightclubs close at a rapid rate with most of us swapping our jägerbombs for piña kale-ada's, the fitness club scene continues to soar and Another_Space is at the heart of the action. Their high-powered HIIT class offers a fast and furious mash up of cardio and strength training with boxing on bags to send endorphins soaring and keep the metabolism firing for hours.

If you like to work on your boxing technique, choose the Boxing Tec 15 / HIIT 45. With all the moody lighting, dramatic instruction on the mic and theatrical shadows from boxing bags, you'll feel like you're about to go on stage... They also offer a dynamic yoga class in the hot room and Primal Vinyasa. A seamless blend of yoga, plyometrics and animal movements. As well as the standard downward dog, you'll find yourself crawling like a bear, even balancing like a flamingo.

The class is designed for anyone looking for a fun, new challenge. If you like an emotionally-charged ride, head for the spin studio and go on a musical journey from Hip Hop to Pop, Garage to House. After working up a sweat, shower off with Cowshed products and hit the on-site cafe for a made-to-order smoothie. Or pay a visit to Farm Stand on Drury Lane, Wild Food Café in Neals Yard or for something a little more indulgent, try The Ivy Market Grill.

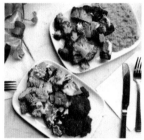
@wearefarmstand

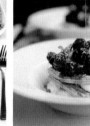
@theivymarketgrill

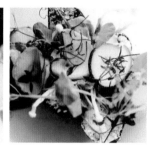
@theivymarketgrill

📍 **Address:** *4-10 Tower Street, Seven Dials, Covent Garden, London, WC2H 9NP*

🚇 **Tube:** *Covent Garden (Piccadilly)*

Notes

....

....

....

....

....

....

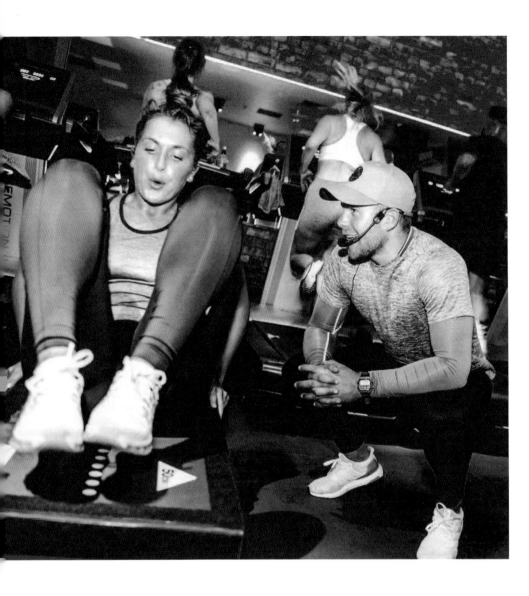

BEST'S BOOTCAMP

HIIT

The half-treadmill, half-strength training routine is a tried and tested formula worth its weight in gold - and even better if you can charge your phone in the locker while you work out. Aside from the spacious shower and changing facilities (stocked with fluffy towels and GHDs) the pièce de résistance is the ice-cold airstream shower designed to bring the body temperature right down post-class. Handy if you have evening plans...no one likes a sweaty date! As for the workout - heart pumping cardio one minute, strenuous strength work the next. Thanks to multiple screens you can keep an eye on your instructor at all times to make sure you're doing the moves correctly (not just copying the person in front of you) and you're always in reach of equipment needed for the class, so not a second is wasted. If you're on the go, grab a salad box or wrap from LEON on the Strand (5 minute walk), or if you fancy a tipple, head to London's oldest drinking den, Gordon's Wine Bar, that offers a great selection of organic, biodynamic and vegan wine and er, cheese! Other options include Covent Garden Grind and LAO Cafe.

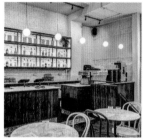
@grind

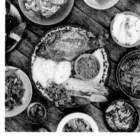
@laocafelondon

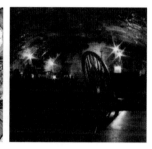
@gordonswinebar

Address: *Concourse Level 1, Embankment Pl, London, WC2N 6NN*

Tube: *Charing Cross (Bakerloo & Northern lines)*

Notes

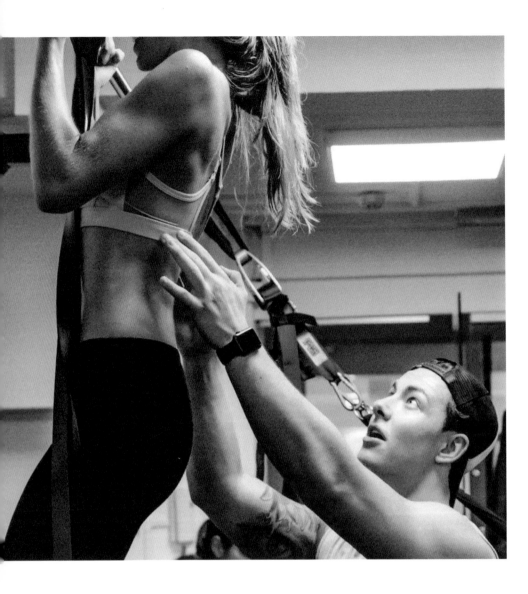

F45 TCR

HIIT | CARDIO | CIRCUITS

Hailing all the way from Australia, F45 burst onto London's fitness scene with its highly addictive group training programme: 27 different workout experiences, carefully curated to ensure class-goers become leaner, faster and more agile. Classes include 'Pipeline', a gruelling cardio workout that's sure to send your heart rate soaring for the full 45 minutes. Work your way around different stations from spin bikes, battle ropes to burpees, box jumps, sandbags and medicine balls. There are a couple of water breaks in-between where you can take a much needed moment to catch your breath before you go all over again. With so much to remember, it's easy to feel overwhelmed but there are two expert trainers on hand to assist throughout, as well as screens playing videos demonstrating each exercise as you work. Yes it's hardcore and you'll be dripping in sweat, but working in such close proximity to others means you can have a laugh whilst taking comfort in the fact you're all going through it together! Afterwards head over to Black Sheep Coffee or BOBO Social.

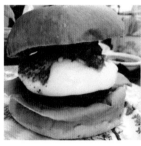 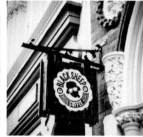 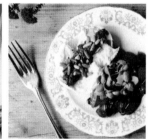

@bobosocialcharlottestreet   @black_sheep_coffee   @bobosocialcharlottestreet

Address: *114-115 Tottenham Court Road, London, W1T 5AH*

Tube: *Goodge Street (Northern)*

Notes

....

....

....

....

....

....

....

....

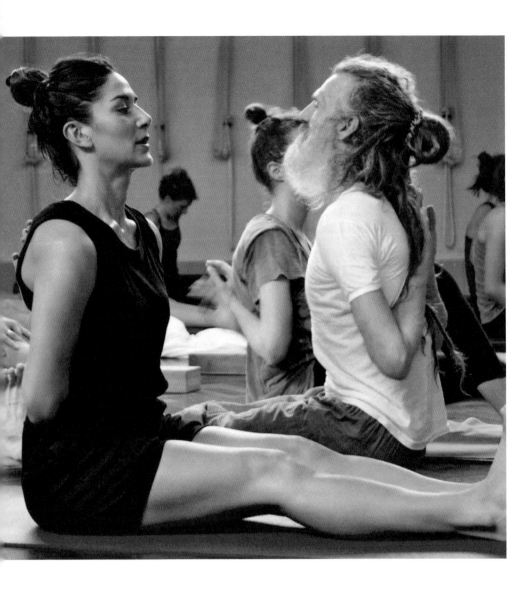

INDABA YOGA

YOGA | MEDITATION

One of London's most loved yoga studios with some rocking teachers and a strong community of dedicated yogis. Discover a range of yoga styles suited to every stage of the yoga journey from beginners and alignment-based classes for those starting out, dynamic and hot yoga for those looking to break a sweat and restorative classes for those looking to unwind and chill. Or if you want to master the art of breathing they run Pranayama classes. Try Yogasana with Stewart Gilchrist (the one with the distinctive dreads and Scottish accent!) known throughout London for his fast-paced, fiery classes with banging beats. Be prepared for a vigorously invigorating Vinyasa flow that's deeply physical and spiritual to leave you with a major high. For healthy eating nearby, you're a 20-minute walk from The Good Life Eatery on Marylebone Lane and the Hemsley & Hemsley café in Selfridges. Or try the Turie cafe and The Mae Deli.

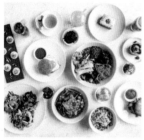 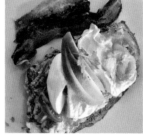 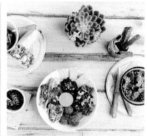

@hemsleyhemsley   *@turiecafe*   *@goodlifeeatery*

📍 **Address:** *18 Hayes Place, Marylebone, London, NW1 6UA*

🚇 **Tube:** *Marybone (Bakerloo) or Baker Street (Bakerloo, Jubilee)*

Notes

....

....

....

....

....

....

....

....

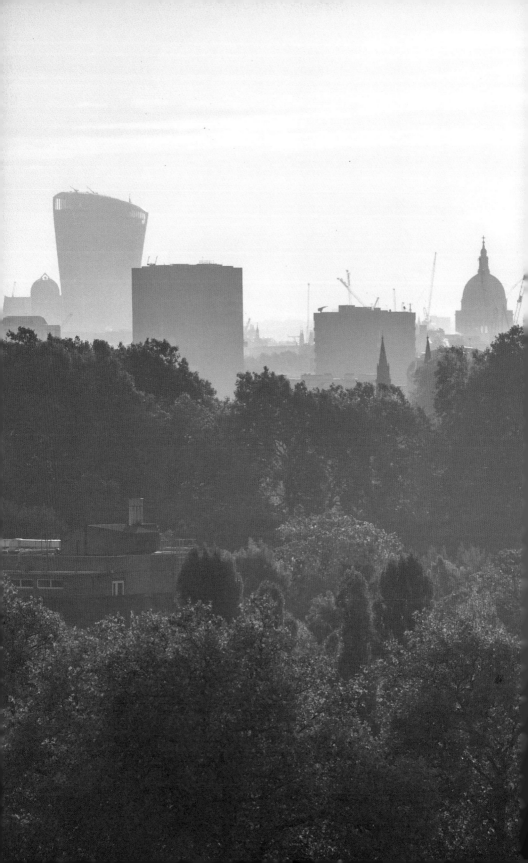

NORTH

*Float above the chaos of the City chasing the
endorphin rush in a nightclub-style studio, find
stillness with candlelit Yin, or sculpt and tone on a
reformer... with a skinny benedict, melt-in-the-mouth
steak and gluten-free pizza to keep you going.*

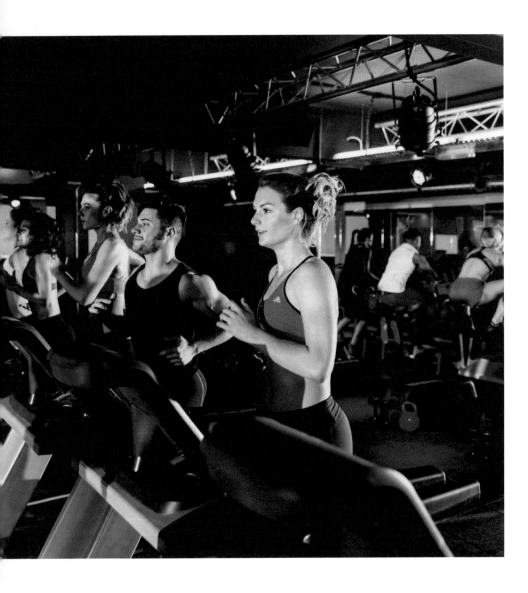

CENTRIC: 3 TRIBES

INDOOR CYCLING | STRENGTH | HIIT

Mix it up with high-intensity interval training, yoga and barre or indoor cycling at this hybrid fitness experience in North London. Try the 50-minute HIIT-style Warrior class - a mash-up of running on a treadmill with the lights down low and a weights section on the floor to a pumping playlist. They also throw in some TRX to keep things interesting. Classes vary between Full Body, Push (arms, back and chest) Pull (legs, bums and tums) and TRX (using your own body weight). If you're a fan of indoor cycling, try Rider, where you'll pedal to beats with choreographed dance, jumps, sprints and hand-held weights. Book your bike online and ride in the high-intensity, low-impact, full-body cycling amphitheatre. Each ride is between 45 and 60 minutes. Or if you're ready to unleash your inner athlete, ride in a Peloton class and compete against yourself and other riders. For post-workout refreshment be sure to pay a visit to Cafe Beam, Irvin Bar & Grill or The Haberdashery for leisurely brunch fare.

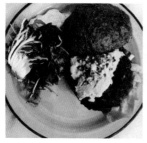 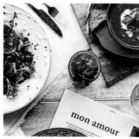 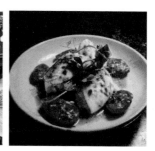

@haberdasheryldn   @cafebeam   @irvin_bar_grill

 Address: *Exchange House, 71 Crouch End Hill, London, N8 8DF*

Tube: *Crouch Hill (Overground)*

Notes

....

....

....

....

....

....

....

....

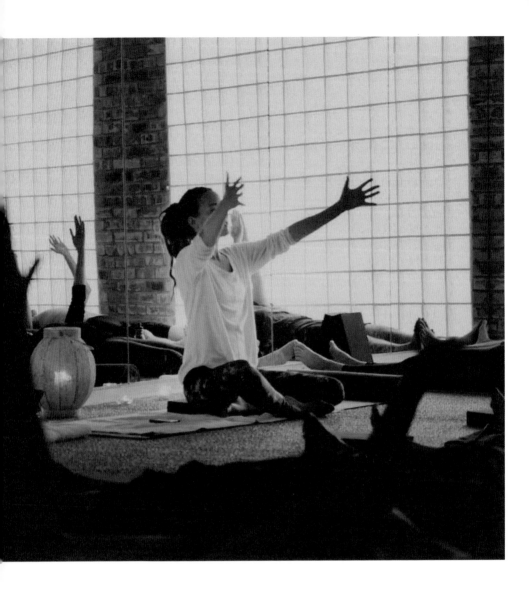

YOGA CENTRIC

HOT YOGA

Ever wondered how North London mums manage to stay so calm and maintain a radiant glow while rocking bodies of twenty-year-olds despite the terrorising toddlers in tow? If you're thinking of packing your bags and heading for nappy valley anytime soon, be sure to learn their secret and discover this gem of a studio. Hot Yoga classes (offered with music or without) range from

60 – 90 minutes with a deep, slow set of movements to re-align, strengthen and de-stress the body and mind. Influenced by Bikram, Power Yoga and Ashtanga, classes are open to all levels. We recommend Sunday's 8.30pm Hot Candlelit Yin class to help you wind down from the weekend or any class with Victoria Grove... the mix of her playlists and voice creates a truly memorable class. For post-yoga refreshment be sure to swing by Ginger & Mint for a cold-pressed juice, Nickel or Coffee Circus.

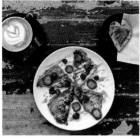
@coffeecircusn8

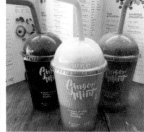
@gingerandmintuk

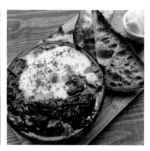
@nickel143

📍 ***Address:*** *52 Coleridge Rd, Crouch End, London, N8 8ED*

🚇 ***Tube:*** *Crouch Hill (Overground)*

Notes

....

....

....

....

....

....

....

....

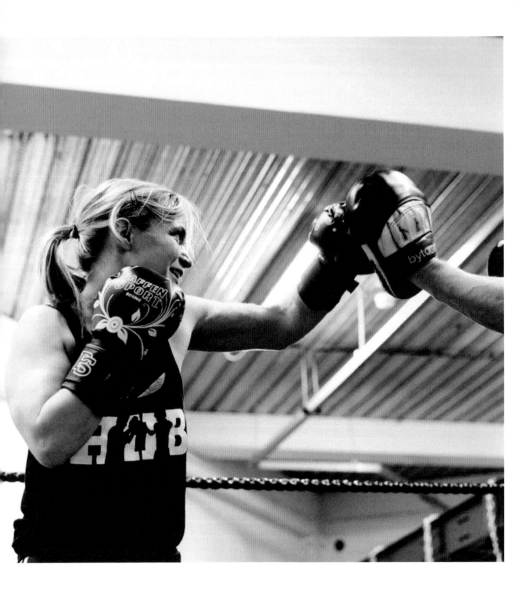

TOTAL BOXER

BOXING

A five minute walk from Hornsey station lies Total Boxer, a technical boxing gym where the idea is to Get FIT Not HIT. Founded by boxing coach Matt Garcia, Total Boxer is one of London's original boxing boutiques. Since the launch in 2012, the club has amassed such a loyal following that classes max out almost instantly. Try a 60-minute Get FIT Not HIT class (if you can get in...) and be guided through a tech check to master your stance, guard, punches and movement, skipping to practise footwork and shadow boxing for technique. While the class bashes away at the bags, you'll be invited into the middle for some one-on-one pad-work with a professional coach. Finish off with some hardcore boxer-style circuit training full of burpees and ab crunches. If you've mastered the basics try FightReady, an advanced boxing session with technical drills and optional low-contact touch-sparring. Or give BoxingYoga a go to kick some serious asanas. There are shared changing rooms, toilets, lockers and shower rooms. To refuel afterwards, head to Edith's House or Heirloom.

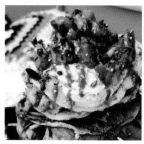
@edithshouselondon

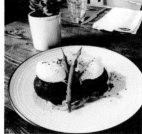
@heirloom_london

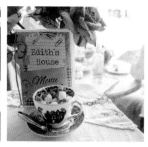
@edithshouselondon

📍 Address: *Total Boxer, 21 Cranford Way, London, N8 9DG*

Ⓣ Tube: *Hornsey (Great Northern Train), Crouch Hill (Overground)*

Notes

....

....

....

....

....

....

....

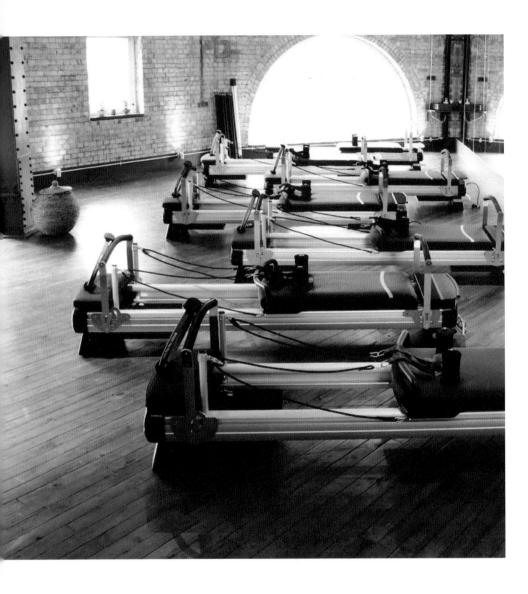

HEARTCORE

PILATES | INDOOR CYCLING | TRX | BARRE | YOGA

The home of London's Dynamic Pilates, Heartcore is seen as the leader of the boutique fitness revolution. Find two studios in North London in St John's Wood and Hampstead. Try their signature class on the custom CoreFormer that will sculpt your physique in ways that traditional exercise simply cannot match. All levels are welcome – though it's a real test of coordination at the start, getting to grips with those straps and springs. Prepare to hoist limbs into all sorts of compromising positions and discover muscles that you never knew you had. Other classes on offer include barre, yoga, indoor cycling and TRX. The Hampstead studio floats above the tube station and is a two minute stroll from fail-safe brunch spot Ginger & White who offer an all-day breakfast menu packed with delicious options like smoked salmon and eggs. If you need something quick and easy, swing by Joe and the Juice on Hampstead High Street. Over in St John's Wood, take part in a fun and powerful TRX class with Gok (a real-life superhero), before paying a visit to healthy hangout Good Life Eatery for a Skinny Benedict. Or treat yourself to something more indgulent at The Ivy Cafe. Lobster scrambled eggs anyone?

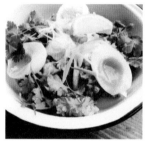 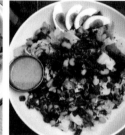 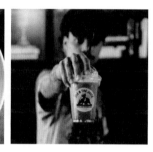

@gingerandwhitelondon   @goodlifeeatery   @joeandthejuice

📍 *Address: Heartcore Hampstead: 50 Hampstead High Street, London, NW3 1QG. Heartcore St John's Wood: 6EA, 27a Queen's Terrace, London NW8*

🚇 *Tube: Hampstead (Northern) St John's Wood (Jubilee)*

Notes

....

....

....

....

....

....

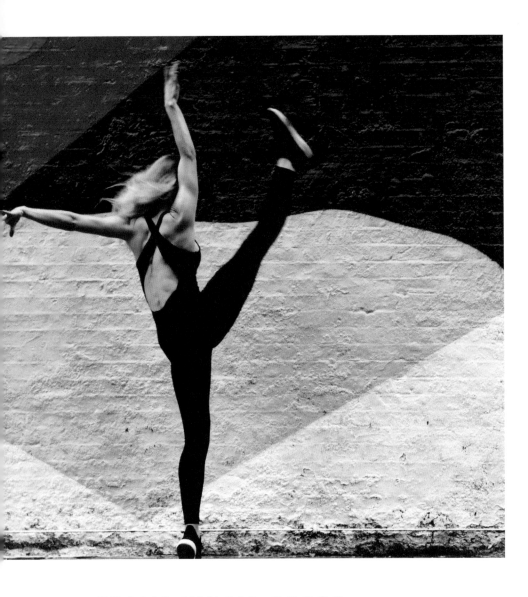

FRAME KING'S CROSS

DANCE | FITNESS | BARRE | YOGA | MEDITATION |
PRE & POST NATAL | PERSONAL TRAINING | PILATES

Once home to some of London's "less desirables", now a stomping ground for fitness lovers who like to brunch and blow-dry post Pilates. Frame King's Cross is a one-stop-shop for all things health and fitness offering everything from strength training and Pilates (with ten thigh-sculpting reformer machines) to a dedicated studio for yoga. Located a one-minute stroll from the main facility, the independent yoga studio offers a range of classes from restorative Meditation and Yin to more dynamic Vinyasa and Rocket. They also run specialised sessions for beginners, mums and sportspeople plus a diverse range of workshops covering everything from inversions and backbends to chakras and acro yoga. The yoga studio has three changing areas but if you fancy a shower, head to the main building with power showers and all the necessary bits and bobs. There's also a shop covering all your wellness needs from activewear and natural skincare to essentials like...spiralizers. Forgot your kit? They've got you covered literally, hire for just £5. You can hang out at their very own Fuel at Frame Cafe that serves protein pancakes and bowls, super-shakes and Caravan coffee. You can also order your fresh juices and shakes before class and find them waiting for you when you're finished. If you want a change of scene, head to Granary Square. The canalside heart of King's Cross home to Granary Square Brasserie, Dishoom, Granger & Co, Maple & King's and Caravan.

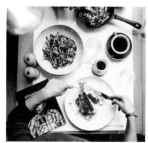 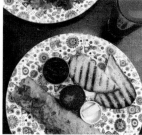 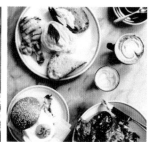

@caravanrestaurants   *@dishoom*   *@grangerandco*

 Address: *ArtHouse, 1 York Way, King's Cross, London, N1C 4AS*

 Tube: *King's Cross St Pancras (Circle, Piccadilly, Hammersmith & City, Northern, Metropolitan and Victoria)*

Notes

....

....

....

....

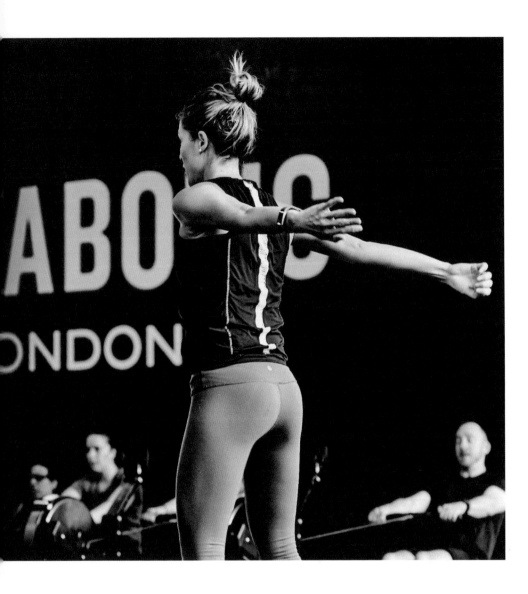

METABOLIC LONDON

STRENGTH | HIIT

The first studio in London to introduce a class dedicated to rowing. Meta-Row, a low-impact, cardio interval workout on the rower mixed with strength and conditioning drills, is one of five classes to launch at Metabolic London. A functional training concept located inside Greater London House, a large art deco building next to Mornington Crescent station. This studio has stripped back all the fancy equipment and nightclub vibes to reveal a basic, rough and ready training space equipped with kettlebells, plyo boxes, rings, battle ropes, sledges and rowers. Classes are designed to build strength, strip fat and burn up to 1,000 calories per session. Try 'Metabolic Signature' – a 55-minute blast of HIIT and strength exercises. Or if you're looking for a quickie to squeeze in your lunch hour, try 'Quick HIIT' – a 30-minute lunchtime smasher designed for time-poor Londoners. Other classes include; 'Meta Circuit' comprised of classic old-school gymnasium circuits to keep the body guessing and 'Viking Method' – a full body workout focusing on building power, speed, strength and agility. For post-workout fuel head to Leyas Coffee or walk 10-15 minutes to Camden Market for vegan burgers at Young Vegans and Korean-inspired Burritos at Kimchinary.

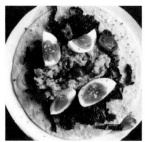
@kimchinary

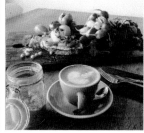
@leyascoffee

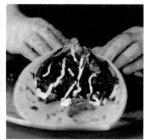
@kimchinary

📍 *Address: Greater London House, Hampstead Rd, London NW1 7FB*

🚇 *Tube: Mornington Crescent (Northern). Camden Town (Northern)*

Notes

....

....

....

....

....

....

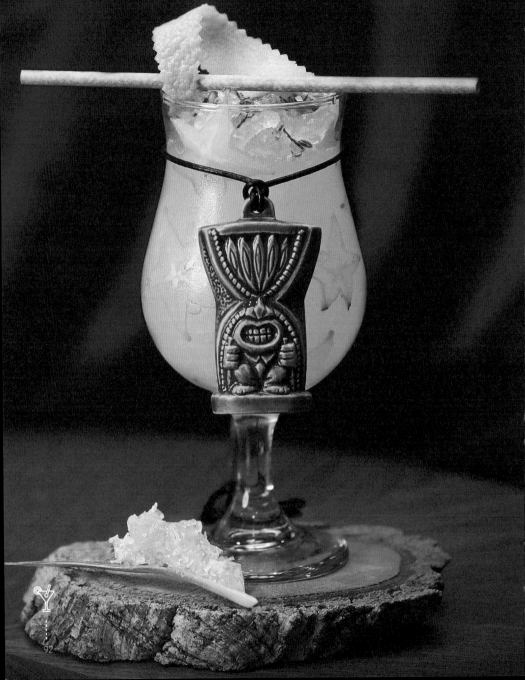

LAKI KANE

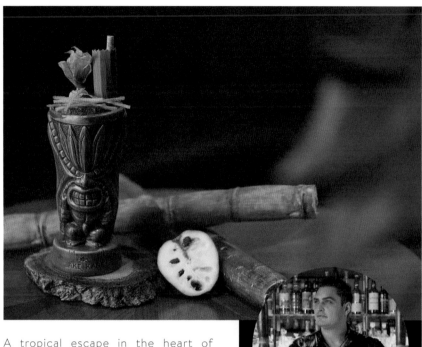

A tropical escape in the heart of London. Be transported to a paradise of entertainment, exploration and the world's finest cocktails. Drinks are freshly prepared using artisanal rums, hand-made sugar cane syrups and sun-ripened exotic fruits, without using any refined sugar.

Tip: Venture upstairs to the Spiced Dry Rum Club to create a special twist on your own personalised rum.

📍 **Address:** *144-145 Upper Street London, N1 1QY*

🚇 **Tube:** *Angel (Northern)*
   Highbury & Islington (Victoria)

Georgi's Laki Kane House Cocktail

Bacardi Cuatro
Chocolate Vodka
Soursop tea
Guanabana
Cupuasu
Fresh sugar cane juice

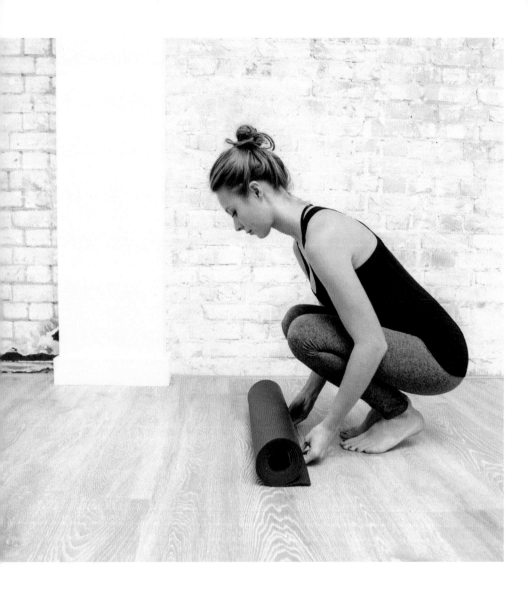

STUDIO I ISLINGTON

HIIT | YOGA | MEDITATION

A bright, airy minimalist studio flooded with so much sunlight, it's hard to believe it was once a dark and dingy karaoke bar. Located on Caledonian Road, a short walk from King's Cross and Highbury & Islington, this is the go-to studio for City workers in search of a balance of high-intensity training and mindfulness. Try their 'Studio One Method' classes, that do just that in one hit. Other classes include: 'Lazy Sunday Yoga', 'Candlelit Yoga' 'Barre', 'Method' classes, 'Yin & Yang Yoga' and reformer Pilates classes. If you've had a tough week and need to calm a busy mind, be guided into a state of deep peace and relaxation in a restorative yoga and meditation class at 4pm every Sunday. It's also a great way to wind down from the weekend. This studio offers sell-out retreats every month aimed at promoting mindful living through a combination of high-intensity training and mindfulness over 3 hours. For dining options in the area, head to Zia Lucia near Highbury & Islington for some guilt-free pizza with vegetable charcoal and gluten free bases, Sunday Cafe or Trawler Trash. There's also a Pret A Manger nearby for something on the go.

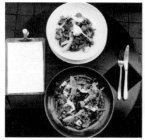 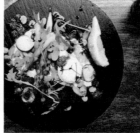 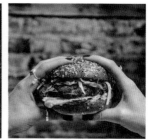

@sundaybarnsbury   @sundaybarnsbury   @trawlertrash

 Address: *237 Caledonian Road, London, N1 1ED*

Tube: *Caledonian Road (Overground) , King's Cross St. Pancras (Northern, Piccadilly, Circle, Hammersmith & City, Victoria)*

Notes

....

....

....

....

....

....

....

ST~GERMAIN

St-Germain is the world's first artisanal French liqueur made with fresh elderflowers, handpicked once a year in late spring. St~Germain is a natural liqueur made with only fresh elderflowers and has no artificial flavor, artificial colouring or preservatives. The classic serve is the St-Germain Spritz: St-Germain, sparkling wine, sparkling water and a lemon twist. The St-Germain Spritz is a light and refreshing cocktail, perfect for brunch or as an aperitif, and is easy to pair with food.

St~Germain Spritz

40ml St~Germain
60ml dry sparkling wine
60ml sparkling water

Fill a tall Collins glass with ice. Add Champagne first, then St~Germain, then Club Soda (the order is essential). Stir completely and garnish with a lemon twist.

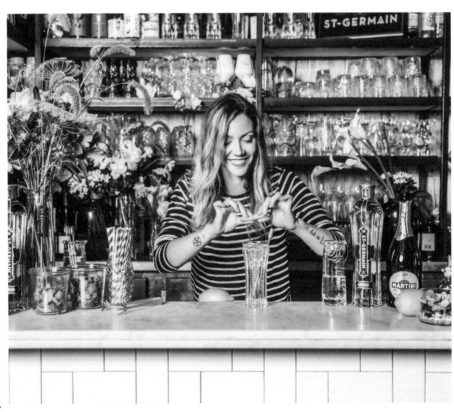

MINT GUN CLUB

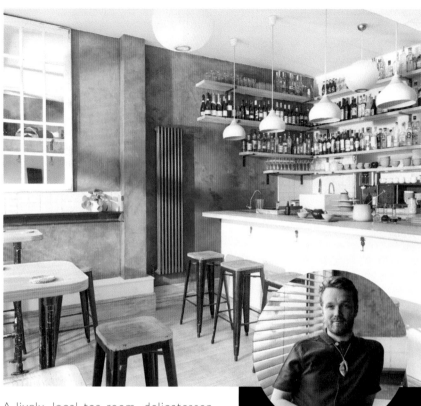

A lively, local tea room, delicatessen and apéritif bar, serving up lassis and kombucha alongside gimlets and coconut wine. It takes its inspiration from the exotic enchantment, elegance and convivial excitement of an adventurous, expatriate lifestyle. **Tip:** *Booking a party? They can accommodate 8 - 70 people.*

Address: *Mint Gun Club, 4a Brooke Rd, London N16 7JN*

Tube: *Stoke Newington*

Rudie's Gimlet

15mls Shiso Cordial
25mls Wray & Nephew
10mls St~Germain
15mls Mineral Water

Stir over ice and serve straight up in a super cold glass. Or add 10% water and pop it in the freezer for half an hour and drink it without the hassle.

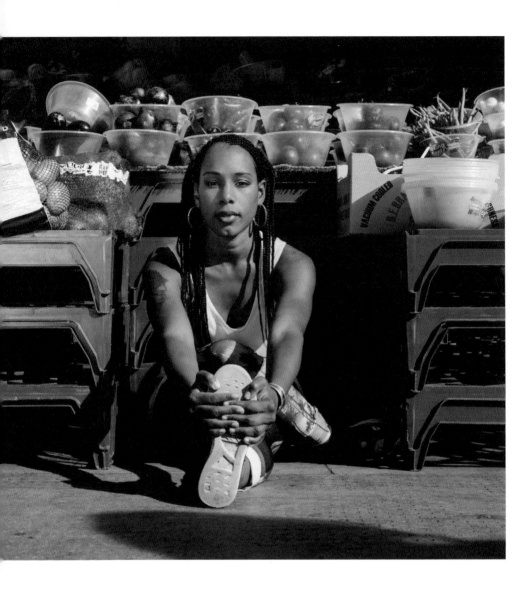

FIERCE GRACE NORTH

HOT YOGA

'We Will Not Om You'. This is no-nonsense hot yoga for the typical Londoner. Find no gongs and oms or preachy 'holier than thou' vibes here – just-to-the point, dynamic stretching in the heat. There's something immensely satisfying in sweating out your sins, contorting the body into positions it could never achieve at room temperature and wringing out organs until they're clean as a whistle - so you can do last night all over again. There are classes to suit a range of abilities from the advanced yogi to S.O.B (stiff, old and broken). Try Fierce Grace, an entry-level class to music full of hip openers, deep twists, upper body strengtheners and bum and ab toners. Wild – a cardio-yoga mash-up with barre, resistance stretching and HIIT. Fierce (aka The Beast) for the hardened yogi or The Fix – a super-charged 50-minute class. For brunch head to Fields Beneath or Arancini Factory Cafe. For an evening affair, pay a visit to Beef & Brew for steak, charred broccoli and sweet potatoes. They have salads, brunch and vegan options too! Carry on the party at Ladies & Gents cocktail bar round the corner.

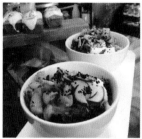 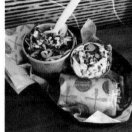 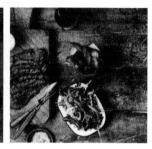

@fieldsbeneath *@arancinibrothers* *@beefandbrew*

📍 **Address:** *173-175 Queen's Cres, Belsize Park, London, NW5 4DS*

🚇 **Tube:** *Kentish Town (Northern)*

Notes

....

....

....

....

....

....

....

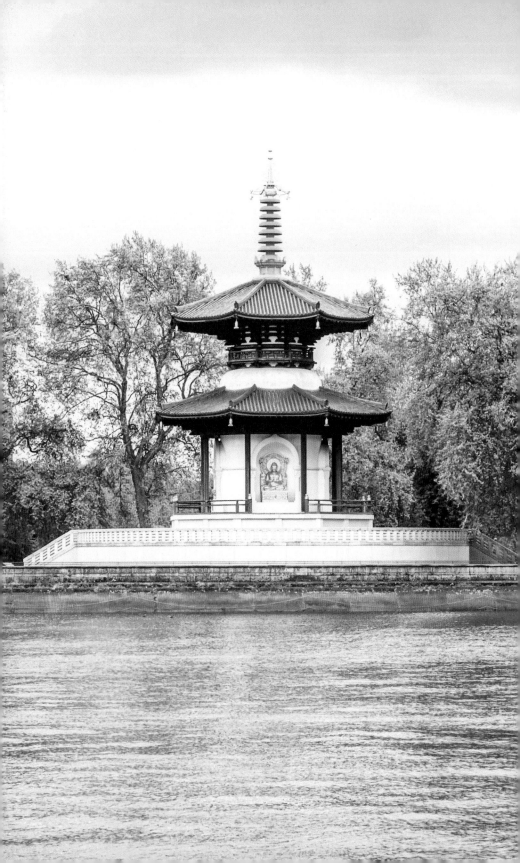

SOUTH

Put your circus skills to the test at an aerial fitness school or try a team-orientated circuits class in Borough before strolling round its legendary food market... do a downward dog above the clouds, discover a fitness party in a clubbing institution in Elephant & Castle, and a lakeside café in Battersea Park...

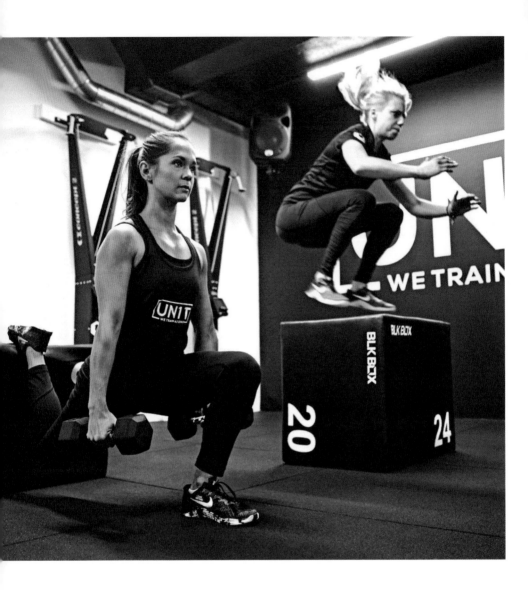

UNIT LONDON BRIDGE

HIIT | CIRCUITS

If you're a fan of team-oriented, competitive training, look no further than UN1T. Encourage, motivate and push fellow comrades to get out of their comfort zones and train as one. As soon as you enter the doors you'll be treated like an athlete and pushed to achieve your best. Try 'Grind' - a mix of cardio movements using bodyweight and equipment with quick transitions between stations for minimal rest time. Or 'Trooper' - a circuit with a competitive twist where the aim is to bank as many laps as possible. A 'Super Trooper' complimentary smoothie is awarded to that one student who pushes that bit harder. All the more reason to go the extra mile. Shower off and head to Flat Iron Square on Union Street for a culinary adventure. Try Where the Pancakes Are - a healthier creperie that uses guilt-free, gluten-free alternative ingredients to cut the unnecessary sugar and stodge! Head to Bar Douro for Portuguese cuisine or Cantina Carnitas for Mexican street food.

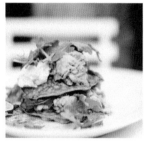
@wherethepancakesare

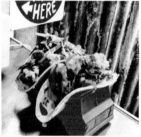
@cantinacarnitas

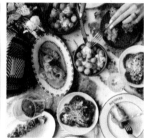
@bardouro

📍 **Address:** *140-148 Borough High St, London, SE1 1LB*

🚇 **Tube:** *Borough (Northern), Southwark (Jubilee), London Bridge (Northern)*

Notes

....

....

....

....

....

....

....

....

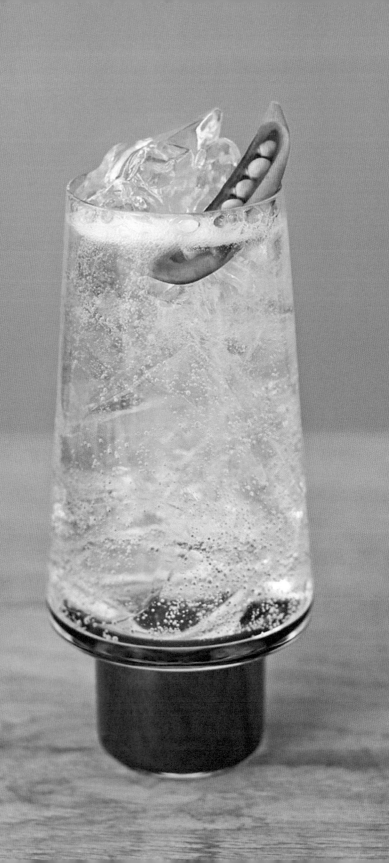

DANDELYAN

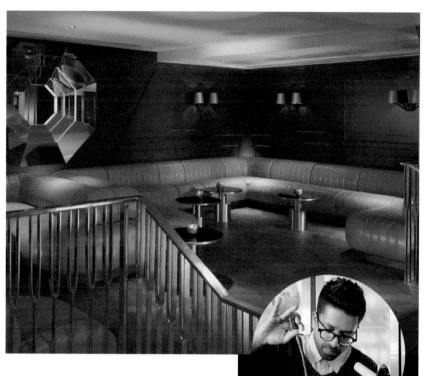

A swanky cocktail bar with pink banquettes, a green marble bar and river views, in a hotel setting. Created by multi award-winning bartender Ryan Chetiyawardana A.K.A Mr. Lyan, Dandelyan plays a mix of late 70s and early 80s rock, funk and disco with top DJs at the weekends, and hip hop for the Sunday wind down.

📍 **Address:** *Dandelyan, 20 Upper Ground, South Bank, London SE1 9PD*

🚇 **Tube:** *Southwark (Jubilee)*

Seedlip Garden 108 & Tonic

Seedlip Garden 108
Fever Tree tonic
Ice
Sugar Snap Pea

Fill a tall glass with ice, add 2oz of Seedlip Garden, top with tonic and then garnish with a sugar snap.

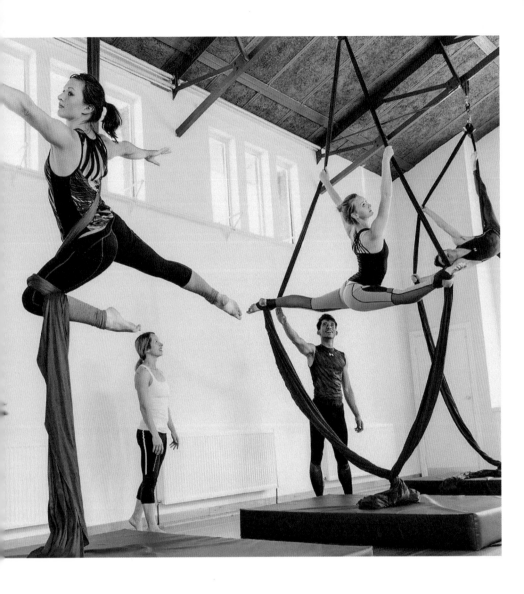

FLYING FANTASTIC

AERIAL FITNESS

Whether you're an aspiring circus performer or first-time flyer, test your strength, stamina and flexibility at this Aerial Fitness School. The super cool venue beneath a railway arch is kitted out with everything any budding aerial fitness fanatic could wish for including a vertigo-inducing 9m ceiling! Experiment with a range of apparatus from hoops to straps, guided by an aerial extraordinaire throughout. They make it look super easy but believe us, it's not. We recommend going with a group of friends and who knows, maybe one of you will turn out to be a born acrobat? Bring a sense of humour and expect to come away with a few aches and pains – you'll discover muscles you never knew you had! Reward efforts in Flat Iron Square, a treasure trove of culinary delights including Tatami Ramen, Savage Salads and Ekachai.

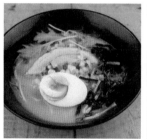
@tatamiramenlondon

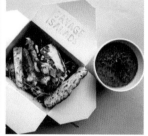
@savagesalads

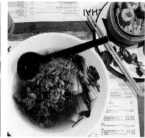
@ekachai_uk

Address: *Arch 27, Old Union Street Arches, 229 Union Street, London, SE1 0LR*

Tube: *Southwark (Jubilee), Borough (Northern)*

Notes

....

....

....

....

....

....

....

....

ST~GERMAIN

St-Germain is also known for its versatility, often considered a 'salt and pepper' ingredient for bartenders.

The cocktail creation possibilities are endless, from adding a dash to a classic Gin and Tonic or glass of Champagne, to pairing with any spirit including vodka, rum, whisky or tequila.

St~Germain
Gin & Tonic

40ml Gin
20ml St~Germain
Tonic Water
2 Lime wedges
Garnish with fresh basil

Fill a highball glass with ice.
Add gin and elderflower liqueur,
and top with tonic water
Garnish with a slice of lime

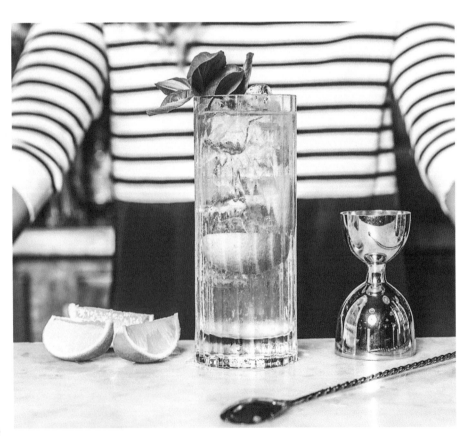

NINE LIVES

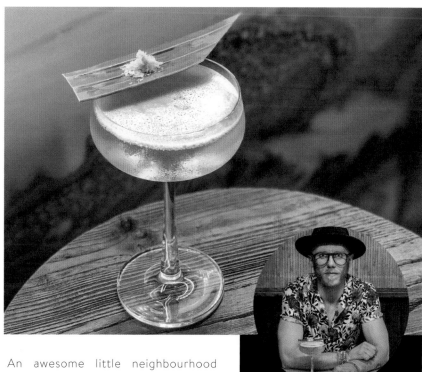

An awesome little neighbourhood bar in Bermondsey Street. This hidden gem, nestled in the Victorian basement of No.8 Holyrood St, is packed full of incredible cocktails, great vibes and a killer soundtrack. Drinks are designed by Tom Soden and the team at Sweet & Chilli.

Tip: Every Saturday they host a weekly party at Nine Lives.

Address: *Nine Lives, Basement, 8 Holyrood Street, London SE1 2EL*

Tube: *London Bridge*

AIKO Cocktail

30ml St~Germain
25ml Fino Sherry
10ml Umeshu
50ml Champagne
1 dash of Grapefruit Bitters
1 pinch of sea salt

Shake, strain & top Coupette

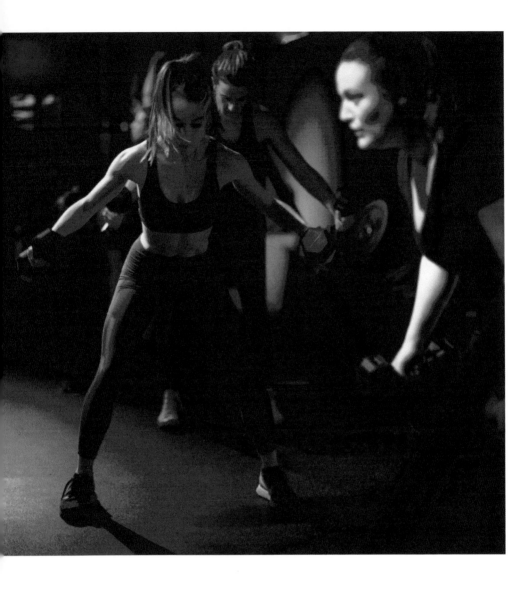

MINISTRY OF SOUND FITNESS

HIIT | CIRCUITS

London's first fitness nightclub. Previously a hidden booze vault, now an immersive HIIT studio, credited with the world's best sound system. Known as Ministry of Sound's fitter sister. The studio is made up of 7 workout stations featuring a wide selection of versatile equipment including self-propelled treadmills, kettlebells, weights, TRX and benches, which are all used in full body combination to test and challenge. Every workout and curated playlist is completely different to the last. With 26 years of clubbing expertise and music knowhow, playlists have been specially curated to get you the best results possible. This is a studio for real people. Posters on the walls actively ban perfect gym-selfies, and as for dress code, no one cares! The club itself often joins forces with legendary instructors for immersive fitness experiences. Afterwards head to Mercato Metropolitano for a delectable feast. Grab a juice from Ginger & Mint or visit Tiny Leaf, London's first organic, vegetarian, zero waste restaurant, for breakfast tacos and eggs with avocado and tomato salsa. The market is also home to some tasty, homemade Vietnamese street food, chargrilled and sashimi red tuna from the Mediterranean, pizzas, tacos and more. Your evening sorted - basically!

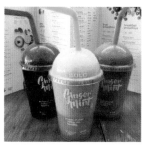
@gingerandmintuk

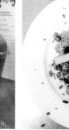
@tinyleaflondon

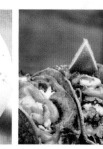
@hermanostacohouse

📍 **Address:** *Arches 80 and 81, Newington Court, London, SE1 6DD*

🚇 **Tube:** *Elephant & Castle (Bakerloo, Northern), Borough (Northern)*

Notes

....

....

....

....

....

....

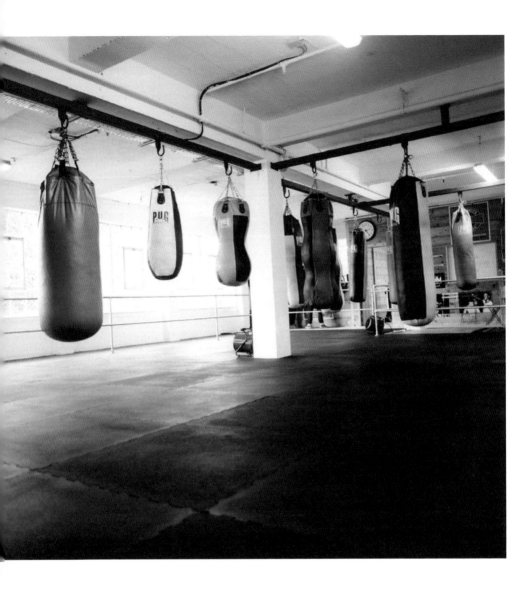

ROONEY'S GYM

BOXING

Master your jabs, hooks and uppercuts at Rooney's - a raw and very real boxing gym in Elephant & Castle. Expect boxing-style fitness classes where you can get a sweat on, while learning how to actually box. What was once an intimidating boxing club under some arches on Bermondsey Street is now a revamped, less frightening boutique gym, floating above a trendy urban farmers'

market. A sure sign of this area's growing gentrification. Before paying a visit to 'The Best Pizza Maker' from Naples... hone your boxing skills first. And we don't mean fannying about doing star jumps next to a bag and hitting it every now and then... Find a mix of skills, bag work, HIIT and killer core sessions in the ring, led by professional boxers and former commonwealth champions. The majority of classes are non-contact and fitness based, with white collar and women's sparring classes for the more advanced. And don't worry, you can still wash and blow dry your hair afterwards. It would be rude not to visit Prezzemolo e Vitale, the legendary independent fresh supermarket from Palermo in Mercato Metropolitano. There's some sizzling steak and sweet potatoes with your name on it too.

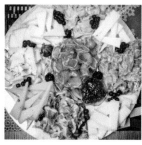
@prezzemoloevitale

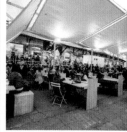
@mercatometropolitano

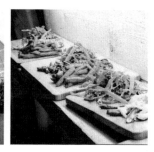
@mercatometropolitano

📍 **Address:** *Rooney's Boxing Gym, Mercato Metropolitano, 42 Newington Causeway, London SE1 6DR*

🚇 **Tube:** *Elephant & Castle (Bakerloo & Northern), Borough (Northern)*

Notes

....

....

....

....

....

....

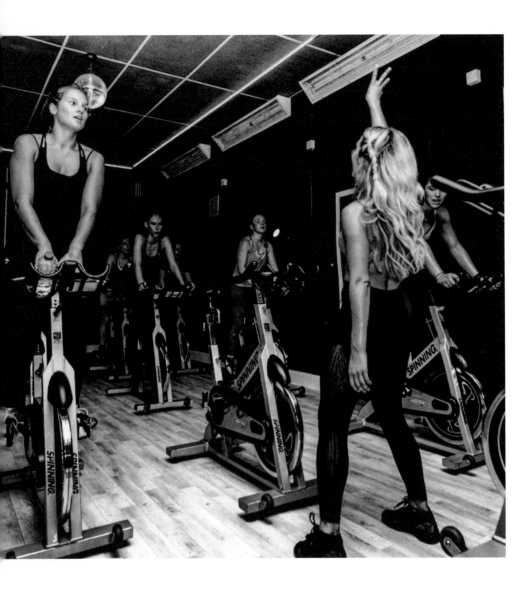

DOG HOUSE FITNESS

BOXING | INDOOR CYCLING

You know that feeling when you're 'in the dog house' after a 'ruff' night? Whether you've disgraced yourself at the staff party or forgot to put the dishwasher on before you went to bed, don't worry, we've all been there. Rather than feeling sorry for yourself, sweat out your sins with a high-energy spin or boxing class instead. Dog House is the go-to destination for fitness, health, and wellbeing south of the river. The self proclaimed "social destination" encourages locals to work, sweat and mingle under one roof. Hence the wine and dog friendly policy. Afterwards grab an 'Abs of Steel' smoothie from Pitch coffee, a mix of almond butter, banana, chia seeds and almond milk. For brunch, head to MILK (though be prepared to queue), Foxlow Balham or if you prefer a cosy pub with a roaring fire, head to The Devonshire.

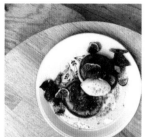
@milkcoffeeldn

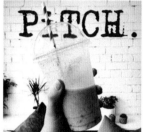
@pitch.coffee

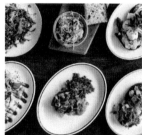
@foxlowrestaurants

Address: *1 Holbeach Mews, Balham, London, SW12 9QX*

Tube: *Balham (Northern)*

Notes

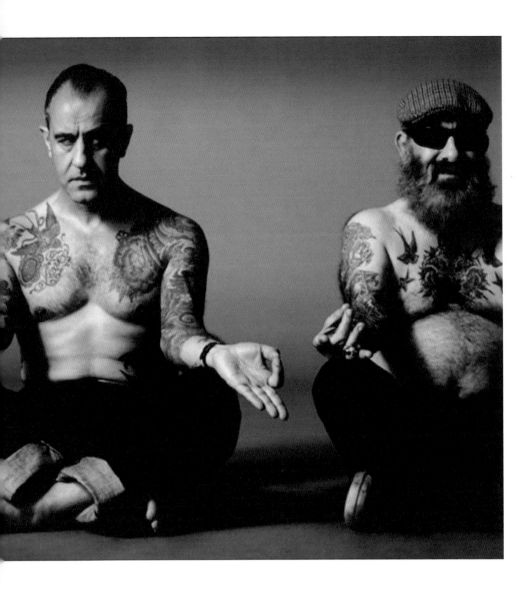

FIERCE GRACE BRIXTON

HOT YOGA

Before you let yourself loose in Brixton Village, practise some discipline inside the Fierce Grace yoga studio. Their challenging user-friendly general level class is full of hip openers, bum toners and moves to test upper body strength and core stability for a fully rounded workout. We're a fan of the Deep Core Candlelit class every Sunday and Monday evening. A deep, slow session that is designed to open you and de-stress you on every level. It's also a great way to work off a hangover. For something quick and dirty, choose the 'Fix' - a 50-minute express class that whips you into shape faster than you can say 'Namaste'. After working up quite a sweat, you'll be relieved to find showers at this facility. To replenish energy levels try a healthy crepe at Senzala, or if Champagne and charcuterie is your thing (we don't blame you) head to Champagne + Fromage. Just remember to hydrate! If you're a fan of grilled Piri-Piri garlic prawns and chargrilled steaks head over to Brixton Village Grill - a bustling Portuguese-influenced restaurant.

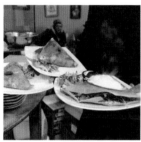
@senzalabrixton

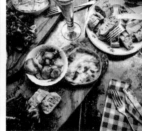
@champfromage

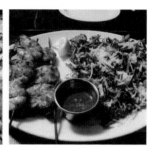
#brixtonvillagegrill via

📍 **Address:** *Fierce Grace Brixton, 372A Coldharbour Ln, Brixton, London SW9 8PL*

🚇 **Tube:** *Brixton (Victoria)*

Notes

....

....

....

....

....

....

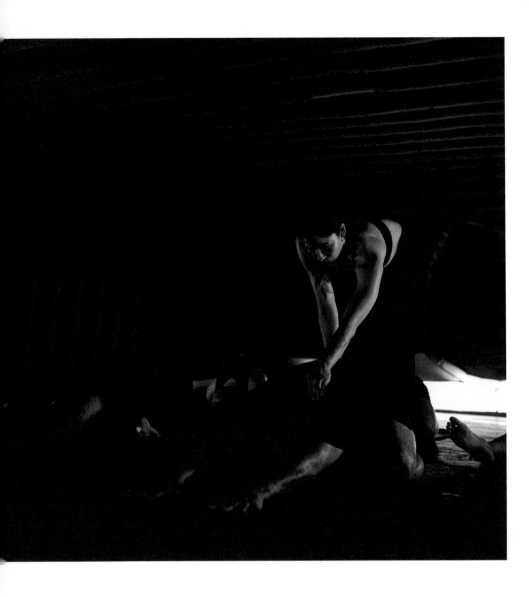

HOTPOD YOGA BRIXTON

HOT YOGA

While permanent Hotpod Yoga homes can be found throughout the UK, South Africa, Netherlands, Portugal and Romania, pop-up versions can inflate just about anywhere from the Austrian ski slopes to music festivals. Today, you can settle with Brixton, Hotpod Yoga's third permanent pod in London (the other two are based in Notting Hill and Hackney). Enter through a bright, spacious reception area where you can hire towels, buy a bottle of water and store your belongings. There are even a couple of showers on site if you fancy making dinner plans. With the pod zipped shut, you'll be transported to another world guided by dim lighting, hypnotic scents and downtempo beats. The 37 degree heat certainly helps you to melt into postures but feels nowhere near as hot as Bikram. If you're left dripping in sweat, hop in the shower and head back to the station – via a leisurely stopover in Brixton Village of course. For a coffee shop and shared work space head to Caya. Or why not treat yourself to dinner at Naughty Piglets, though you'll be feeling more like a smug little piglet after an hour in that pod. Just remember to pack a towel and a big bottle of water!

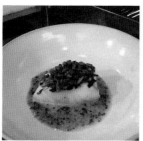
@naughtypiglets

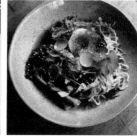
@salon_brixton

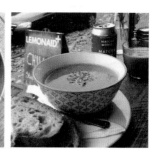
@caya_club

Address: *40 St Matthew's Road, Brixton, London, SW2 1NL*

Tube: *Brixton (Victoria line)*

Notes

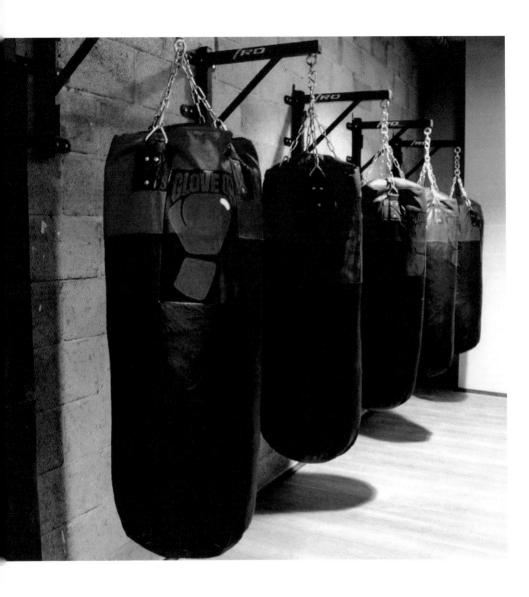

GLOVE UP

BOXING

There's boxercise and there's boxing. If you're a fan of the latter with genuine kit and quality instruction (with people who know what they're talking about), visit this gem of a studio that offers everything from Thai Boxing to Kettlebell Circuits. In memory of Martin Holgate, the founder of this gym, this is what Glove Up is all about: "Glove Up is the attitude and approach to life and the adversities it throws at us. In all our lives there is a moment where we are presented with the choice of giving up, curling up in the corner and conceding defeat or fighting back. Glove Up is to choose to fight back." Try a Boxing Fitness Conditioning class with John Tiftik - expect a dry sense of humour and an intense mix of boxing and circuits to improve technique and overall fitness, open to all levels. Boxing gloves and wraps are provided for no extra fee and there are showers on site. Located fifteen minutes from East Putney or ten minutes from Wandsworth Town, try a Saturday morning class and refuel at Brew for a post-workout breakfast or brunch. For evening plans try Ben's Canteen or The Ship.

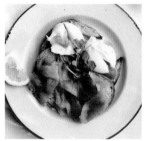 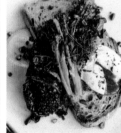 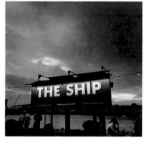

@brew_wandsworth   @benscanteen   @theshipwandsworthimnotafiend

---

📍 **Address:** *22 Hardwicks Square, London, SW18 4GS*

⊖ **Tube:** *East Putney (District) or Wandsworth Town (South West Trains)*

Notes

....

....

....

....

....

....

....

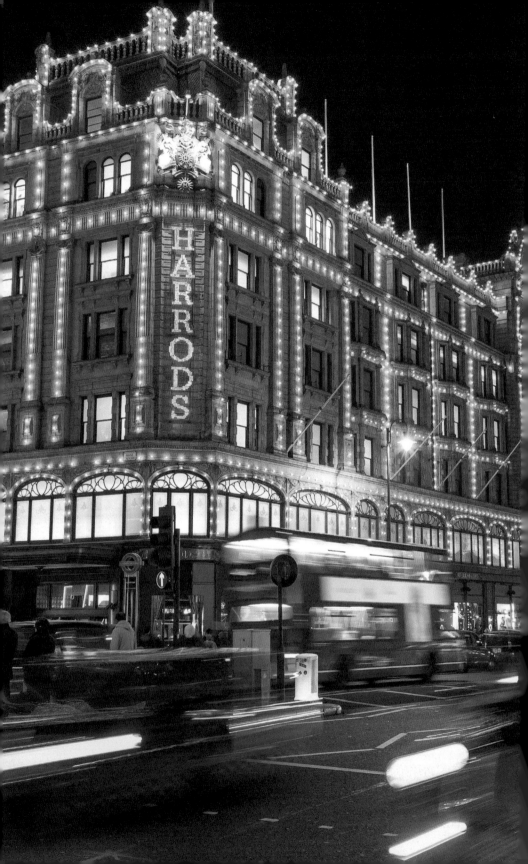

CHELSEA & FULHAM

Chase your workout with a session in an Infrared sauna or cryo chamber and discover a boxing gym that's more nightclub than Fight Club in Sloane Square... discover the meaning of 'barre to bar' in Fulham.... and park your pram in the crèche before indulging in a spot of bouncing and brunch in Parson's Green.

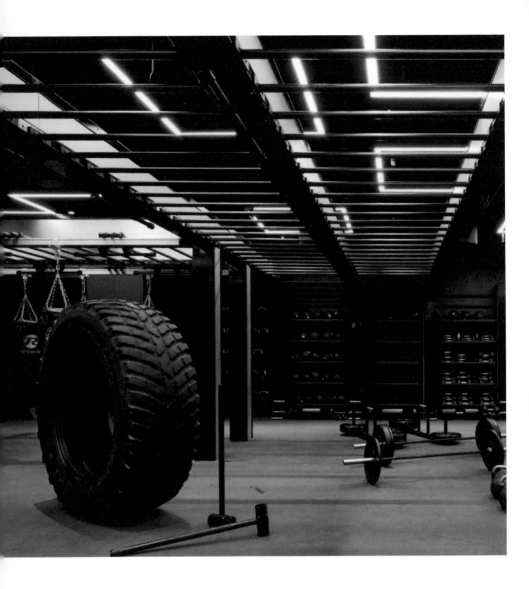

KXU

INDOOR CYCLING | BARRE | STRENGTH BOXING | YOGA

The pay-as-you-train version of KX, a 4 minute walk from Sloane Square station, offering a range of classes from HIIT & Run, NOK OUT to Paola's Body Barre. You can even pay a visit to an infrared sauna (aka "microwave" sauna for how it heats the body from within), or freeze your assets in a Cryotherapy chamber. If you like your spin class to feel more like a house party in a darkened room with disco lights with a sound system to rival Glastonbury try U-Cycle. For a mighty metabolic conditioning circuit try Meta-K, or if you're looking for a gentle, friendly flow book Vinyasa yoga. Need to unleash the beast? Try The GAMES - a strongman-style circuit, complete with sledge hammers, sleds and tractor tyres. Top it off with an LED facial and lymphatic pressotherapy ... (it's all in the add-ons here!) Post workout head to Raw Press for a juice or grab a salad box to go at Baker and Spice. Other foodie delights in this area include Orée, Dominique Ansel's Bakery, L'eto Cafe and Raw Pressco. For something fancy head to Restaurant Ours in Knightsbridge.

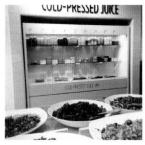
@rawpressco

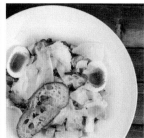
@letocaffe.co.uk

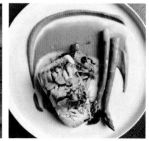
@restaurant_ours

Address: *241 Pavilion Rd, Chelsea, London, SW1X 0BP*

Tube: *Sloane Square (Circle & District)*

Notes

....

....

....

....

....

....

....

....

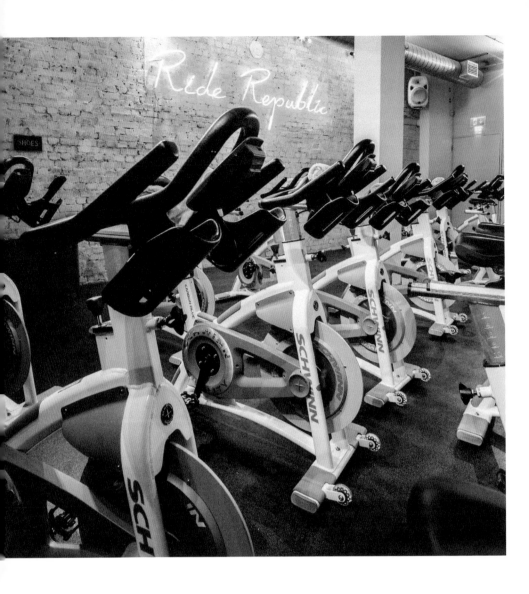

RIDE REPUBLIC

INDOOR CYCLING

A boutique indoor cycling realm in Fulham, offering high-intensity low-impact rides in a neon-lit studio. The built in burn board system projects your live score onto a screen for everyone to see to spur on a spot of friendly competition. It's not just your legs that get blasted – they also incorporate arm and core exercises to help tone your whole physique. Try 'cardio & core' that includes one extra track for flexing the muscles and a 10-minute bolt-on of tummy-toning exercises on the floor. If you're strapped for time, try 'Burn Express', an efficient 30 minute class to squeeze in your lunch hour, with a complimentary smoothie or coffee to take back to the office! The team will prepare your bike just for you in advance every time you ride and cycling shoes and towels are provided for all rides. There are also lockers, showers and Bamford bath and body products all on the house! For some post-workout refreshment, take a 15-minute stroll to Rude Health serving nutrient-dense, cultured and fermented natural foods. Try the weekend brunch menu with healthy treats like Avo on Toast with Poached Eggs and Sprouted Spelt Pancakes! Other options in this area include Boys'N'Berry and Gail's Bakery.

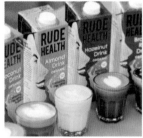 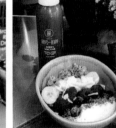 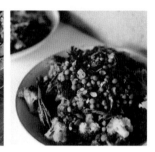

@rudehealthcafe   *@boysnberry_london*   *@rudehealthcafe*

📍 **Address:** *709 Fulham Rd, Fulham, London, SW6 5U*

🚇 **Tube:** *Parsons Green (District)*

Notes

....

....

....

....

....

....

....

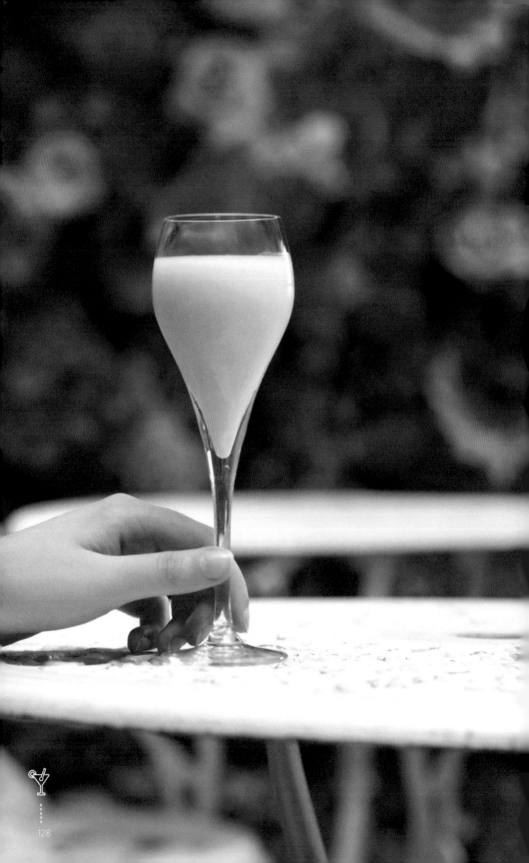

BARTS

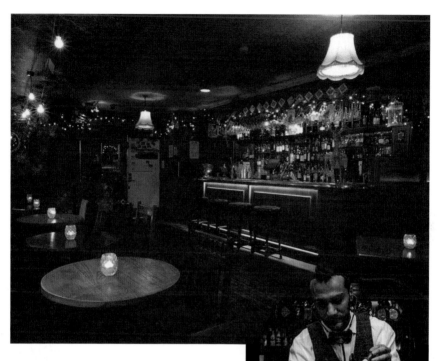

A speakeasy cocktail bar set in the 1920s prohibition era, run by Chicago gangsters, with quirky wall ornaments, dressing-up boxes, and a vintage afternoon tea. If you know the password, the door is open from 6pm 'til late every day. Barts serves the finest yet most illicit liquors.

Tip: Book a Criminali Tea every Sat at 2pm and try The Secret Garden.

📍 **Address:** *Chelsea Cloisters, Sloane Ave, Chelsea, London SW3 3DW*

🚇 **Tube:** *Sloane Square*

Birch Better Have My Money

Freya Birch spirit, Avocado syrup Lme juice Dill and walnut oil

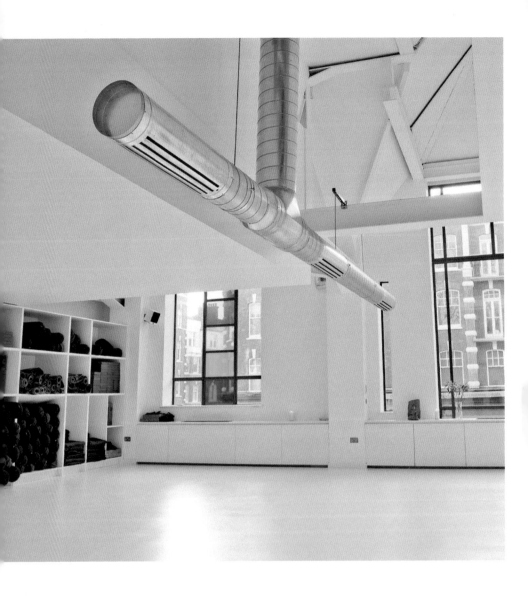

TRIYOGA CHELSEA

YOGA | PILATES

Following its launch in Primrose Hill, Triyoga quickly became the go-to yoga studio of A-listers including Gwyneth Paltrow and Kate Moss. This centre on the King's Road offers three studios, three treatment rooms, an organic café and a juice bar. Find every conceivable type of yoga from Ashtanga to Vinyasa, hot yoga to Kundalini, Iyengar to Yin.

They also offer a range of barre, Pilates and Gyrotonic classes plus an ever-evolving programme of workshops with resident gurus. The idyllic yoga sanctuary also offers a range of treatments from deep tissue massages to acupuncture and craniosacral therapy. Founder Jonathan Sattin's vision was to offer great teachers and authentic styles of yoga in a gorgeous uplifting environment where yoga could be accessible to everyone – regardless of age, size, gender, fitness, diet and lifestyle.

Today there are five centres located in Soho, Camden, Chelsea, Covent Garden and Shoreditch. After your class, peruse the latest athleisure in the shop and swing by the organic café and juice bar. Head to A Wanted Man for healthy wholesome food and artisan coffee or Rabbit for fresh farmed and foraged seasonal fare. For a decadent brunch in lush surroundings, head to The Ivy Chelsea Garden.

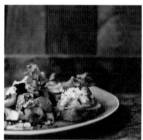
@awantedmanlondon

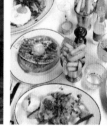
@ivychelsgarden

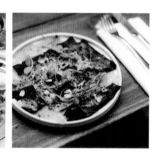
@ rabbit_resto

📍 **Address:** *372 King's Rd, Chelsea, London, SW3 5UZ*

🚇 **Tube:** *Sloane Square (District & Circle)*

Notes

....

....

....

....

....

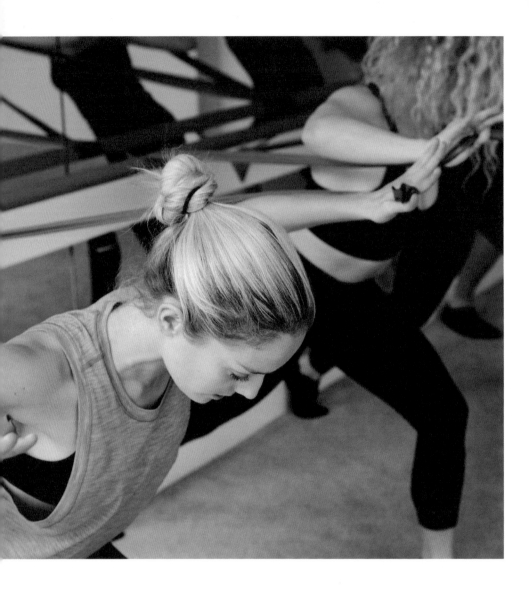

BARRECORE CHELSEA

BARRE

Recognised as London's original barre studio and now with studios in nine locations across London, Barrecore fuses the moves of ballet, Pilates, yoga and functional training. Classes include their SIGNATURE class, a low-impact, full-body interval training programme using isometric exercises alternated with stretches to create a long, lean physique. Or, if you prefer your workout to have more of a yoga vibe, try ASANA. It incorporates signature Barrecore moves with restorative yoga poses. This fast-paced, flowing class will challenge you physically and energise you mentally. Alternatively, if you want to crank it up some more, try the SCULPT class with resistance bands for that added intensity! After all that sculpting, shower and head to London's cult healthy food joint, The Good Life Eatery, for a Skinny Benedict, Joe & the Juice, or Waitrose for a grab-and-go salad. For something a little more fancy head to Tom's Kitchen, the brainchild of award-winning chef Tom Aikens for Baked Turkish Eggs, Sweetcorn Fritters and Turmeric and Matcha Lattes.

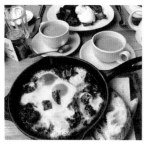
@tomskitchens

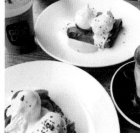
@goodlifeeatery

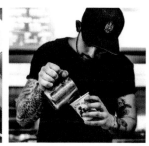
@joeandthejuice

📍 *Address: Barrecore Chelsea, Atlantic Court, 77 King's Road, First Floor, London, SW3 4NX*

🚇 *Tube: Sloane Square (Circle & District)*

Notes

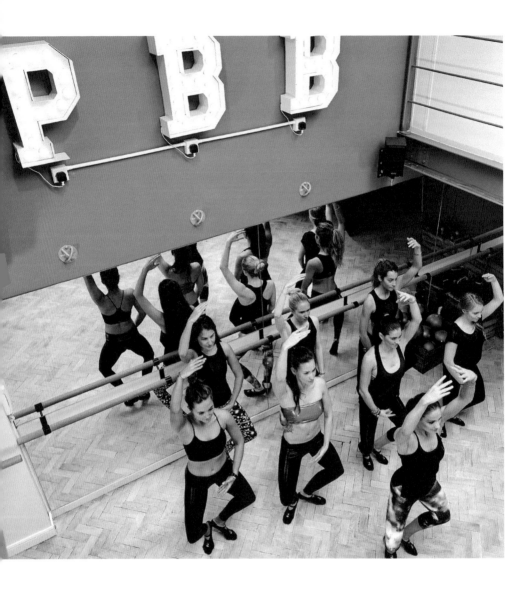

PAOLA'S BODY BARRE

BARRE

Popular with the Made In Chelsea set, Paola's Body Barre method draws on elements of Pilates and ballet barre techniques with jaw-dropping results. Her signature method gets into the deeper stabilising and peripheral muscles, working them to exhaustion resulting in tight, chiseled limbs. Try PBB Signature, a dynamic, high energy (low-impact) class to an upbeat sequence that yields incredible results. This is how you craft a tight, chiselled body. After just three or four sessions, you can expect lean limbs, amazing posture and a very strong core! Be sure to bring your barre socks – no trainers required! Looking for something punchier? Try PBB Burn with a focus cardio - upping your heart-rate and feeling the burn, incorporating elements of functional training and bodyweight work. There's also a 45-minute express class if you're looking to squeeze a session into your lunch break. For a cross between fitness and dance try PBB Tone it Up - an upbeat, high-energy, high-intensity class which incorporates dance sequences to get your heart rate up and your sweat on. Other specialist classes include Boxerina® - a fusion of Paola's BodyBarre Method and boxing that will see you go from shadow boxing, kick-boxing to passé into a deep plié! Afterwards head to Glasshouse Coffee, Rude Health, Boma Bridge or Aussie style cafe Antipodea. We promise it's worth the 20 minute walk!

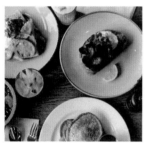 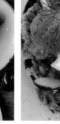 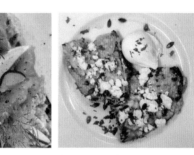

@antipodealondon   @glasshouse.coffee   @bomarestaurants

📍 *Address: Paola's BodyBarre Fulham, 2 Fulham High St, Fulham, London SW6 3LQ*

🚇 *Tube: Putney Bridge (District)*

Notes

....

....

....

....

....

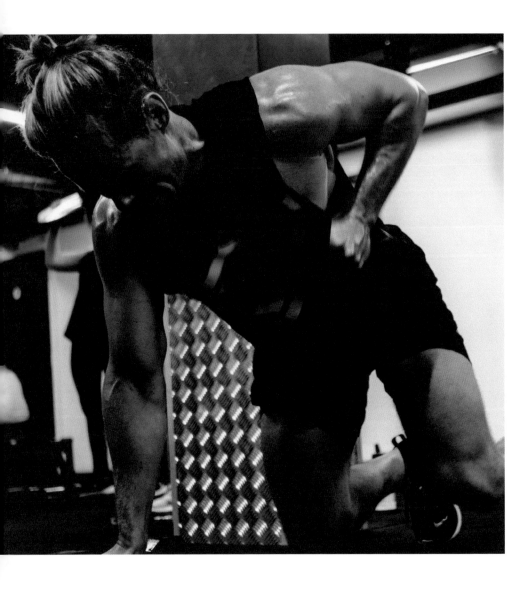

UNIT

HIIT | CIRCUITS

A high-octane, tabata-style workout next door to Joe's Brasserie. Earn your eggs benedict with relentless rounds of circuits to boost athletic performance. Located inside a basement warehouse with exposed metal pipes, find a high energy crowd and a DJ at the decks. Try the ENTITY class with circuits of ski ergs, TRX jumps, mountain climbers and burpees. Race down an astro track on all fours and hurl medicine balls. A non-stop battle of endurance that will leave your heart racing – fast. Buddy up and perform each exercise twice for 20 seconds with 10 seconds' rest in-between – then repeat the circuit 3 times. You'll be grateful for a cool down on the Air Dyne Bike – like your very own wind machine to transport you into a JLO video. Finish with a deep stretch and help yourself to foam rollers and trigger point therapy balls for a spell of active recovery. There's also 'Yoga For Un1t's' every week to help you balance out. Shower off and afterwards, head to Joe's Brasserie or walk 15 minutes across Wandsworth Bridge to The Ship - not your average London pub.

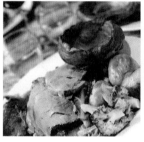
@theshipwandsworth

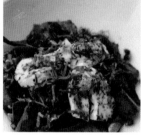
#joe'sbrasserie

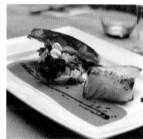
@theshipwandsworth

📍 *Address: UN1T Fulham, 132 Wandsworth Bridge Rd, London SW6 2UL*

🚇 *Tube: Fulham (District), Imperial Wharf (Overground)*

Notes

....

....

....

....

....

....

....

....

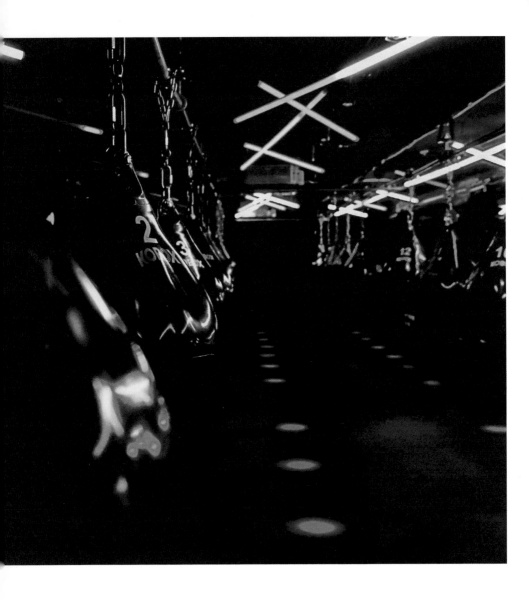

KOBOX

BOXING

A boxing studio that's more nightclub than fight club brooding inside a shopping centre off the King's Road. As the lights dim low and the beat drops, expect to blast all your inhibitions away. Their signature Boxing HIIT workout is split between skipping to activate muscles, 'punch by numbers' on the bags to help you through some mind-boggling combinations and strength training – push ups and pulls ups being their favourites. Expect to slam some medicine balls and be put through punishing rounds of box jumps, resistance work and weights. Each class is designed to torch calories, improve coordination and help you channel your inner badass. First-timers will need to pay for a set of branded wraps on arrival. Make use of the spacious changing facilities and head to Comptoir Libanais for a Lebanese feast of hot mezze and halloumi. You're also a short walk from Daylesford and The Botanist near Sloane Square station. If you're in a hurry, swing by the KOBOX Kitchen that offers protein-packed smoothies, healthy food and snacks.

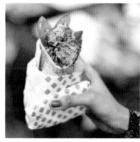 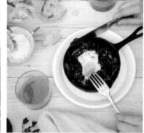 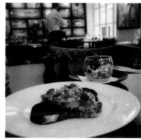

@comptoirlibanais   @daylesfordfarm   @thebotanistsonsloanesquare

Address: 7-12 Sloane Square, London, SW1W 8EG

Tube: Sloane Square (Circle & District)

Notes

ABOUT THIS GUIDE

Every reasonable effort has been made by Whatever Your Dose Limited to trace the copyright holders of material in this book. Any errors or omissions should be notified in writing to hello@whateveryourdose.com. We will endeavour to rectify the situation for any reprints or further editions.

This is a City guide created to help pleasure seeking wellness enthusiasts navigate London's fitness scene.

Cover image "ChromaYoga" by Stephanie Sian Smith
Studio photography provided by venues
Food photography from Instagram (handles provided)
Destination pages: Shuttershock

Created by Hettie Holmes, Editor of DOSE
Graphics by Luisa Inwood (www.lcidesigns.com)

DOSE is an online magazine for healthy hedonists.
Sign up to their newsletters at whateveryourdose.com

Follow @DOSE on Instagram

Notes

11937626R00082

Printed in Germany
by Amazon Distribution
GmbH, Leipzig